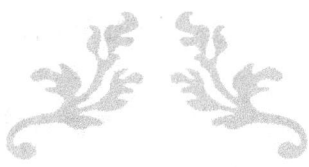

THE PHARMACIST IS A WHORE

How pharmacists lost control of their profession and why you should care

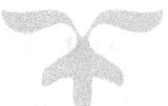

BY KIM ANKENBRUCK RPH

Cover photograph "Raleigh Rye Girl" by E.J. Bellocq c.1912, from his collection chronicling the Prostitutes of Storyville, the legalized red light district in New Orleans from 1897-1917

CHAPTER 1

THE WHORE AT THE CORNER

OF HAPPY AND HEALTHY

Not so long ago, in a far-away land, a little anal-retentive introvert of remarkable intelligence and verbal ability was born. As the little cherub grew, she drew the admiration of every adult who met her with her respectful behavior and pleasing personality. She completed any chore she was assigned without complaint, and she could be counted on to work independently. If need be, she would sacrifice play time to get things done. She excelled in school, bringing home straight A's and glowing comments about how well behaved she was in class. She graduated from high school and went straight on to college, got her BS in pharmacy, and, diploma in hand, went out to seek her fortune.

One day, she met a pretty man wearing a grey pinstriped suit, smelling of expensive cologne and sporting a fresh haircut and manicured fingernails. He showed her a shiny brochure decorated with pictures of a beautiful boat, an expensive car, and lots of golden eggs in a nest. The words "Profit Sharing" were prominently displayed at the top of the page. The pretty man smiled broadly and told her that all these things could be hers if she agreed to work for him, and she signed the offer of employment eagerly.

Her new job was very hard, but she was making lots of money. True, she missed seeing her friends and family in the evenings and on weekends, and sometimes she had to work on holidays to take care of the customers the man sent to her. But she was a professional, and she performed her duties well and without complaint. Sometimes she felt as if the man asked too much of her, and sometimes he asked her to do things that didn't seem right. Some of the customers asked her to do things that weren't right, either, and it was hard for the people pleasing girl to resist giving in to their demands. But for the most part, she could still do the job and stick to her principles, so she made the best of things and soldiered on.

In early September, rumors began to circulate about a terrible flu epidemic brewing in the land. The pretty man came to the girl and told her that she was to be trained to perform a new service, a service that would benefit all mankind. The name of the service was "flu shots", and they would be given all day, every day, without an appointment. Only the best pharmacists in the kingdom would be giving flu shots. Soon, there were so many customers wanting flu shots, the girl could not keep up. She asked the man for more help, but the man said no. He told her that soon she would be asked to give all kinds of shots to more and more people. She would be expected to do all of her other duties while giving these shots. The man said that she was not making him enough money to warrant extra help, and, in fact, he was taking away some of the help she already had, until she proved herself to him.

The girl tried very hard to make the man and the customers happy. On one particularly busy day, the man showed up at the pharmacy with a stack of papers in his hand and shoved them in her face. He told her that he had thought of a new way to make money, and she was going to be pricking the customers fingers and checking their blood sugar and cholesterol. She would be weighing them and taking their blood pressure as well. These papers were to be used to write down the services and bill for them.

The girl began to cry. With these new tasks, she would be truly overwhelmed. How could she do her job properly if she had no extra help? The man said he did not care. He said that there were plenty of other pharmacists who wanted a wonderful job like hers, and that he would have to hire one of them to replace her if she could not keep up. He said that he had heard that her attitude was negative, that she had a short temper, and that she wasn't able do all of the tasks required of her. Maybe she was just getting too old. Maybe she was doing bad things when she wasn't at work. Maybe she wasn't cut out to be one of the elite pharmacists of the kingdom anymore.

The girl had to admit she didn't like herself anymore. She was drinking too much, and she was up all hours of the night worrying about the pharmacy and the customers. She no longer did things with her friends and family, and on the rare occasions she did see them, she treated them badly and spent the whole time complaining about her job.

One day, the girl came in to work as usual, and the store manager told her there was to be a drug test that day, and that no one was to leave the store. The girl was not worried, because, although she abused alcohol, she did not take any medications that were not prescribed to her, and she had been working for the man for 15 years without one positive drug test or write up.

On a Monday morning, two weeks after the random drug test, the pretty man came to the pharmacy and told the pharmacist her drug test had come back positive and she was suspended. He told her to sign her name on a paper that said she was taking the drug that showed up on the test. She objected, but the man made her sign the paper anyway, because if she did not, she would be fired on the spot. After signing the paper, she was escorted out of the store and told not to come back until she could prove she was not taking drugs anymore.

The girl did not know what to do. She had always been a good girl, a smart girl, a straight "A" student and an honest and caring member of society. How could this have happened to her? She considered killing herself, but decided she would take a walk in the park and try to clear her head. When she got to the park, she saw a woman sitting on a bench, smoking a cigarette and closing her eyes as she blew smoke into the warm spring air. She was wearing a shabby purple dress, and her shoes and stockings had seen better days. She wore a huge, floppy purple hat with a downy red feather soaring high into the air and waving in the breeze. The woman took one look at her and knew something was terribly wrong.

"Hey toots, what's got your tits in a ringer? You look like you've lost your best friend or sumptin'."

The girl gave a wan smile and told the woman her story. The woman began to laugh. Soon she was stamping her feet and slapping her knee, and tears were running down her face. The girl was offended and started to leave, but the woman stopped her.

"Now, now, hang on there just a minute, missy. The reason I'm laughin' is because I used to be a pharmacist, and a pretty good one, too. I was doin' all the things the man wanted me to do, and I was makin' money for him hand over fist. Then he decided I was gittin' too old and wasn't makin' enough money no more, and he said he was going to replace me with a newer model. He told me I wasn't working fast enough or filling enough prescriptions. He told everybody that I was pickin' up drugs off the floor and taking them, and that I was stealin' medication from the pharmacy. I got real upset, and I decided to go drown myself in the river. I was sittin' on a bench just like I'm doin' now, when an old lady appeared out of nowhere and sat down beside me. She asked me what was the matter and I told her the whole sad story. It was then that she said the truest words I ever heard, or will ever hear. She looks me right in the eyes and she says to me 'Why, you're nothin' but a goddamn whore!'."

"You can go straight to hell" I says, and I got up quick like and made to get away from that ol' bag. She grabbed my arm and stopped me in my tracks."

"Now hold on, hold on. Listen here. Ain't you said you worked for a pretty man wearin' a fancy suit and tie with an expensive haircut and a manicure?"

I allowed as that was true.

"And didn't you say you was makin' money for the man hand over fist, and he didn't 'preciate it nohow? And didn't you say he kept addin' more and more services for you to perform for the customers, but you wasn't gettin' a percentage of the profits, and you was fit to be tied?"

I allowed that was true, too.

"And he threatened you and tol'you all the time that he was 'gonna' punish you or git someone younger than you that could make him more money?"

"All of a sudden, it begun to dawn on me that the 'ol gal was right. Not only was the fancy man my pimp, and I was one of his whores, I had to be the stupidest whore on the face of the planet, because even a whore gets a percentage of the profits for extra services.

Here I had been breakin' my back workin' and sweatin' and apologizing for my very existence, while he was livin' large with all his fat cat friends, laughin' all the way to the bank.

As long as he could keep me down, he was happy. I let that man say and do things to me I never let any other human being say or do, just so's I could have the PRIVILEGE of working the corner of Happy and Healthy for his benefit."

The girl began to smile for the first time in a long time. "So, what did you do? Did you quit, did you start your own pharmacy, did you work for a hospital or long -term care or mail order outfit?"

"Hell no, girl. I figured since I was so good at prostitutin' myself out anyhow, I might as well go into the business myself and leave out the middle man. My reputation was ruined, my confidence was in the shitter, and I was sick and tired of bein' abused just to make somebody else richer. None of my former pharmacist "friends" would even talk to me, let alone vouch for me. I was poison, you see. I might soil their good name if they associated with the likes of me. Abandoned me just like that, even folks I had known since college. A bunch of goddamned gutless sheep is what pharmacists are. Turn on you the first chance they get, figure they ain't never gonna be in your shoes. But just you wait til that new sheep herdin' pup comes along and starts learnin' the ropes from the old dogs. He's young and hungry, and he's a gonna' push them sheep until they don't know which way is up. One of these days he's gonna drive them sheep right on through the fence and over the cliff out on the back forty, and then they'll be a layin' at the bottom of the hill a cryin' and a squallin' and a wonderin' what the hell happened to their cherry pie life."

The girl felt freer than she had in years. A great weight had been lifted from her shoulders, and she could breathe again. She did not know right then what she was going to do, but whatever it was, she was never going to subject herself to the kind of hell she had been living in for the last 15 years.

    She thanked the old woman and gave her a kiss on the cheek. As she turned to go, the old woman winked at her and said "Darlin' you're gonna be just fine, as long as you respect yourself and never ever lay yourself down for the man."

CHAPTER 2

WHY YOUR PHARMACIST IS A WHORE

I know, I know, but stay with me for a minute. A pharmacist is a "professional" who has a certain set of skills to offer. The district manager is a "pimp" who is backed by a corporation with cash and powerful connections. The corporation sets up the business and finances it, and puts the pimp in charge of the whores. The pimp runs the show, but he also protects his employees, or gives the illusion of protection.

Times are tough, and the pimp isn't making as much money for his bosses as he used to. That's when he realizes his whores have marketable skills that he can exploit for cash. He writes up a price list, with a fee for each service performed, and he makes sure the whores know he means business when he says they must push clients to accept these extra services or else.

He also forces the whores to apply for and obtain a registration number, which allows him to bill clients for services the whore performs. He says it's obvious that the whores won't be getting any of the income, as they are expected to provide the extras as part of their regular duties.

According to mirriam-webster.com, the synonyms for "pimp" are: *Abuse, capitalize (on), cash in (on), impose (on or upon), leverage, milk, exploit, play (on or upon), use, work.*

Related words include: *Jerk around, manipulate, mistreat; bleed, cheat, fleece, overcharge, skin, soak, stick, commercialize, commodify.*

The same source lists the synonyms for "prostitute" as: *Abase, bastardize, canker, cheapen, corrupt, debauch, degrade, demean, demoralize, deprave, deteriorate, lessen, pervert, poison, profane, debase, subvert, vitiate, warp.*

Related words include: *weaken, disgrace, dishonor, humiliate, shame, take down, downgrade, hurt, impair, wreck, ruin.* (Mirriam Webster Dictionary 2017)

In what way does this arrangement not resemble prostitution? When the district manager (aka pimp) comes to visit a store, he arrives in his black, shiny Lexus. His toady, the pharmacy district manager, hops out of the passenger seat. Make no mistake, the DM for the stores is always in the driver's seat. The pimp has a fresh haircut and a manicure, and is wearing a bespoke suit and custom made white dress shirt. His expensive black shoes have a warm glow, courtesy of a shoe shine at the airport on his last business trip. The suit is generally black. The tie may be traditional and stolid, or it may be bright and playful, meant to portray the pimp as a fun and funky hipster, a guy who can do business during the day and party at night. The two men leave a scent trail of expensive cologne and hair product as they breeze through the aisles.

The district manager for the pharmacy follows meekly behind the pimp. He is dressed in similar attire, black suit, white shirt, colored tie, black shoes. He is holding a clip board and jotting down notes. He nods and smiles every time the DM mentions his name or includes the pharmacy in the conversation. He generally does not speak unless spoken to.

Behind the pharmacy DM is the store manager, pandering to the pimp's every comment and whim, eager to please. The tone of the visit is one of friendly camaraderie, but there is a sinister undertone, a feeling that something wicked this way comes. The unspoken thing that underlies every interaction with the DM is intimidation.

The employees know that they must be on their best behavior, and that a wrong answer or comment may make them a target. It is best to say as little as possible, and to agree with every single thing the DM says. The pharmacy manager is expected to drop everything when the DM glides into the pharmacy, shake his hand heartily, smile and nod, and bend over for the next high hard one the DM is set to deliver.

Meanwhile, the bosses at the corporate offices collaborate in their elegant conference rooms, while they consume their catered lunches, hashing out the various and sundry ways they can squeeze more money out of the highly paid professional whores that they are unfortunately required by law to employ to handle their pharmacy business.

The gullible pharmacists perform more and more services with the same resources and for the same pay. What stupid whores they are to continue to enrich the pimps by prostituting themselves for their benefit. The pimps laugh all the way to the bank, collecting outrageous salaries, stock options, and bonuses, while the pharmacists in their employ ruin their physical and mental health and damage their personal lives trying to meet their ever-increasing list of demands with bare bones staffing.

The pharmacists may have sold themselves into prostitution, but they had a lot of help. The schools and colleges of pharmacy indoctrinated their young charges, painting a pretty picture of respect, prosperity, and professional fulfillment, knowing full well that these glowing depictions were lies. They allowed the pimps to come in to their universities and wine and dine the students, luring them with cheap pens and coffee mugs into a dark and dreary life that no one was willing to warn them about.

While this irreverent depiction of the chain of command and operation of the modern retail chain pharmacy may be tongue in cheek, it is nevertheless quite accurate. Although almost no one is willing to talk about these glaring and persistent abuses, any pharmacist who works for a retail chain will tell the same sad tale if you buy him enough alcohol to overcome his inhibitions.

The only person standing between you and complete disaster in the drug store is your harried, hassled, exhausted, anal retentive pharmacist. Contrary to what you may think, these dedicated professionals are on your side. The type of individual who stays in this profession is a perfectionist. They want to help you, but they cannot help themselves. Their bosses hold absolute power over them, and they monitor their every move via hidden cameras, computers, and unscrupulous employees who report back with any infraction. They are faced with the near impossible task of pleasing the tyrant while still providing you with your medication as quickly, accurately, and safely as possible. It is not an exaggeration to say that if not for these dedicated professionals, there would be a lot more injuries and deaths due to medication errors.

CHAPTER 3

AT THE CORNER OF WICKED AND WEALTHY DANGER, WILL ROBINSON

Every time you have a prescription filled, you are putting your life on the line. As a pharmacist, I can tell you that the corporations running chain pharmacies do not care about you or your health. They care about profits and stock prices. With deep pockets and armies of corporate lawyers, the chains are untouchable in a court of law. Millions of dollars in fines and settlements have done nothing to dissuade them from running their pharmacies like poorly staffed fast food joints, as if medications were no more dangerous than burgers and fries.

Dr. Jekyll and Mr. Hyde have nothing on the real-life actors behind the scenes of the big retail pharmacy chains like CVS and Walgreens. Behind the cheery ads, Red Nose days, charity walks, and free Central Park concerts lurks a sinister corporate money grubbing behemoth who cares little about quality of care or patient safety.

"Pay no attention to that monster behind the curtain" the executives croon, smiling benevolently in their press release photos while they conceal the real reasons medication errors are on the rise, and why pharmacists are torn between struggling to meet the demands of their corporate bosses while ensuring the safety of their patients.

While Congress fumbles around with the new healthcare bill that is supposed to replace the Affordable Care Act, patients are being endangered by a healthcare system run by corporations and business managers who only care about the bottom line, and who disregard the needs and opinions of the healthcare professionals who used to be in control of patient care.

As you will see in the following pages, that white coated introvert behind the counter is not your real enemy. Although you may view this person as the "Drug Police", the "Insurance Denier", or the "Smug Smartass" who questions you or your doctor, the truth is, the pharmacist is one of the few people left in this cynical business who actually cares about you and your safety. The demands on today's retail pharmacist are draconian. The unreasonable metrics enforced by retail chain stores compromise not only the health and safety of the public, but the health and safety of the pharmacists and technicians who fill the prescriptions.

Daniel A. Hussar, Remington Professor of Pharmacy at the Philadelphia College of Pharmacy at the University of Sciences in Philadelphia, publishes a monthly newsletter entitled "The Pharmacist Activist". His take on the situation in retail pharmacy is succinct and spot on.

"There are many very capable and highly professional pharmacists working in chain pharmacies, and some enjoy their responsibilities. However, many others do not. Their greatest threat comes from the executives and other decision makers in the

companies in which they are employed. The concerns I hear most often from chain pharmacists pertain to the stressful workplace environment, inadequate staffing (both pharmacists and technicians), very low salaries for technicians, the metrics and the clock (e.g., quotas for the number of prescriptions and immunizations; the number of minutes in which a prescription is expected to be dispensed; the number of rings within a phone call must be answered), no or limited time to speak with patients, the lack of professional fulfillment, and the intimidation of higher managers and a fear of retaliation. These concerns are even greater now than they were just several years ago, because of the tightening of the employment market for pharmacists. Chain pharmacists who have concerns or even constructive suggestions are more reluctant to communicate them to their manager and above for fear they might be putting their job at risk at a time when employment elsewhere may not be available." (Hussar 2014)

CHAPTER 4

THE FALLACY OF MCPHARMACY

Prescriptions are not burgers. The public is understandably unaware of what goes on behind the pharmacy counter, and they cannot be expected to fathom the depth of attention to detail and the thought process involved in filling every prescription. It is not the public's fault that they have been led to believe that preparing a prescription requires no more brains or finesse than assembling a Happy Meal.

Standing at the counter at McDonald's, you can see employees in the back frying burgers, lowering fries into hot oil and sliding them into containers, assembling the completed burgers and wrapping them, pouring drinks, waiting on drive through customers, and helping customers at the counter. In no case will you see one employee performing all of these tasks with no help, yet that is exactly what you will see on a given day in a chain pharmacy. The pharmacist often works alone or with the help of only one pharmacy technician for an entire shift.

If you think a customer is angry when their burger order is messed up, you can multiply that reaction a thousand times when it comes to their medication, and rightly so. Compare the risk of harm between "I said no pickles" and "You gave me heart medicine instead of thyroid pills" and you will understand the insanity of the current pharmacy workplace model.

In December of 2016, the Chicago Tribune published a series of investigative reports which took two years to complete. The Tribune tested 255 pharmacies to see how often retail pharmacists caught their intentionally planted drug interactions and warned the patient of the danger. There were five drug pairs included in the tests, selected with help from pharmacy professors. Each pair represented a classic significant drug interaction that should have been easily caught by the pharmacists. In 52% of the cases, this did not happen. (The Chicago Tribune 2016)

When questioned, the chains hid their dirty hands behind their backs and scuffed the bottom of one shiny black shoe across the ground in a "gee whiz" gesture of false contriteness, promising to retrain their negligent staff, update their computer software, and send out memos emphasizing the importance of checking the patient's profile for drug interactions. CVS even promised to institute a hard stop on computer alerts which in the past could have been overridden by a pharmacist without contacting the doctor. This update required them to call the doctor for each and every issue flagged by the computer.

In other words, the money grubbing SOB's blamed the whole thing on the pharmacists and outdated software. Each and every retail pharmacist wants to scream at the top of their lungs

"It is not training or the lack of another pop up on the computer screen that is the problem, it is your asinine metrics and bare bones staffing, you moral cretins!"

U.S. News and World Report published a similar article back in 1996, sounding the alarm with the headline "Danger at the Drugstore: Too many pharmacists fail to protect consumers against potentially hazardous interactions of prescription drugs". If you read the article, you can see that not much has changed in the 22 years since it was published. (U.S. News Online 1996)

I have been a pharmacist since 1984. During my five years in pharmacy school, we were told that a new era of pharmacy was dawning, and the days of "count, pour, lick and stick" were over. We would soon be delegating those mundane duties to technicians, leaving us more time to engage with and educate patients about their medications. This in turn would allow the pharmacist to use her unique knowledge to increase patient safety and optimize medication therapy. Maximizing medication therapy is a fancy way of saying that it is in the best interest of the patient to provide them with medicine that treats their condition without causing more harm than good, while paying attention to factors like convenience, lifestyle, realistic goals, and cost.

Fast forward to 2018. Not only are we still counting, pouring, licking and sticking, we are also immunizing, performing health screenings (cholesterol, blood glucose, blood pressure, ideal body weight), and conducting appointments for medication therapy management. While we are doing all these things, understand that there is nobody checking the prescriptions, taking prescriptions over the phone, or counseling patients. Only the pharmacist is legally authorized to perform these functions.

There are seldom two pharmacists on duty, and usually only for an hour overlap at the shift change. If the store budget allows, a pharmacy technician or two may be assigned to help fill prescriptions, answer phones, and ring up customers, but the burden of responsibility still rests with the pharmacist. In no case should the pharmacist ever be working by themselves, yet this is becoming the norm in most retail pharmacies.

The chains make the excuse that the store managers can help the pharmacists if need be on days when there are no technician hours available, but this is a joke. Not only do the store managers resent having to help in the pharmacy, a good number of them are completely useless and represent a hindrance instead of a help. Some chains require their store managers to become licensed pharmacy technicians by taking the NHA's CPhT test. This ruse allows the chains to claim there is a pharmacy technician on duty, but, unfortunately, these "technicians" bear little resemblance to the legitimate, experienced technicians relied on by pharmacists.

Even the best technicians do not have the knowledge required to thoroughly evaluate and check a prescription. They receive on the job training, must have a high school diploma, and must pass an exam administered by the State. The pharmacist has either a BS or Doctor of Pharmacy degree, and 5 to 6 years of education. While there are technicians who are extremely competent, they work under the supervision of the pharmacist, and the good ones respect the pharmacist's judgement, perform their duties well, and are a godsend.

If you do a Google search for "workload and pharmacy errors" you will find hundreds of links to articles in magazines and newspapers, as well as links to blogs and forums discussing the problem of pharmacy workload and dispensing errors. (See Appendix for links to pertinent articles). Unfortunately, the corporate goons who dictate the course of our profession do not care that medications can harm and kill people. They continue to apply the fast food assembly line model to the filling of prescriptions, and poorly at that. Ray Kroch would turn over in his grave if he saw the modern prescription filling process applied to the preparation of his beloved burgers.

Nothing pharmacists have tried so far has done anything to change our dangerous working conditions, not the articles, not the blogs, not the books, not the activists, not the pleas to pharmacy organizations and the state boards, not unionization, not the letters and calls to government officials, not even the investigative reports filed by national news teams sent out across the country and viewed by millions of people. Not one of these efforts has made one whit of difference. One can only come to one conclusion. Corporate profits trump safety. Period.

CHAPTER 5

BE WELL

If you think the chains have your best interests at heart, think again. Consider the following:

Pharmacists no longer have any say in how the pharmacy department is run. The district manager, who is not a pharmacist, issues directives from corporate to the store manager, who passes on these directives to the pharmacist in charge (PIC). When and if he visits the store, the Pharmacy District Manager effectively sits on the store DM's lap like a ventriloquist's dummy, spewing out corporate speak, blind and deaf to anything the pharmacists have to communicate. He is no longer one of us.

Executives and middle managers make huge salaries and bonuses, creating a conflict of interest that blinds them to patient safety concerns. The number of pharmacists in these positions have dwindled, leaving the pharmacy in the hands of individuals who chose a business career over a career of service to patients.

Performance metrics encourage pharmacists to take risks and shortcuts. Metrics are statistics used to evaluate how a pharmacy is performing in categories like wait times and time taken to answer the phones. Metrics do not take into account intangibles like time spent counseling patients or giving immunizations. (CVS 2010)

The penalty for ignoring the metrics is staff cuts, reprimands, write ups, and disciplinary action. Metrics can also be used as tools to push out older, more experienced (and more expensive) pharmacists. Troublemakers who point out the dangers of production quotas and skeletal staffing eventually find themselves out of a job.

Pharmacists are expected to give immunizations and perform health screenings and blood pressure checks for patients "all day, every day" without an appointment, despite the fact that they are often the only person working in the pharmacy, especially in the evening and on weekends. Training and giving injections is mandatory, despite the fact that some pharmacists are needle phobic or don't want to deal with blood and needles. The training is minimal and consists of reading through a lengthy booklet (published by ASHP) in one half day session, and taking a test on the booklet the next day. The second day is also devoted to performing ONE intramuscular injection, and ONE intradermal injection in front of the trainer.

Pharmacists are afraid to push for patient safety because they will be targeted for elimination. Pharmacists are pressured, coerced, and threatened with losing their jobs if they make trouble for the managers. Chains use dirty tactics to eliminate "non -team players" who try to voice concerns over workload and patient safety.

Age discrimination is rampant and has become one of the clandestine ways the chains are cutting down on their payroll expenses. Pharmacists over 50 are being fired or pushed out, and new pharmacy grads are being hired at lower salaries and kept below the hours needed to be eligible for benefits. There are plenty of new grads available, since the number of pharmacy schools has escalated in recent years. In 1982, there were 72 pharmacy schools. As of July 2018, that number has nearly doubled.

Another abuse perpetrated by the chains is the lack of 15 minute breaks and 30 minute lunches for pharmacists. Pharmacists are "professionals" and fall under the category of "management", which means that lunch and breaks are not mandated. They often work 12 to 14 hours without eating, drinking, or using the bathroom. This is not an exaggeration.

The state boards of pharmacy, who are supposed to regulate the practice of pharmacy and advocate for patient safety, have been infiltrated by chain pharmacists who use their position on the board to further their employers' interests. When the board is questioned about their obvious and continued lack of action regarding work load and staffing, their traditional response is "we are not in the business of telling employers what to do". The attorneys general who oversee the state boards of pharmacy are similarly closed mouthed on the subject of working conditions in retail pharmacy chains, and their impact on patient safety.

Unionization has been put forward as the only way to combat the problems of poor working conditions, at will employment, unpaid overtime, staffing levels, sick time, and maintenance of seniority by legacy pharmacists. Some pharmacists think unions will create more problems than they solve, and they cannot square the concept of walking off the job with the responsibility they have to their patients. This is why professionals like pharmacists, nurses, and teachers have traditionally avoided unions, and their employers take advantage of that integrity.

CHAPTER 6

IT'S A SHITTY JOB, AND YOU HAVE TO DO IT

Everybody thinks their job sucks. I get that. We all think that if we won the lottery we would be happy, fulfilled, and at peace. It is hard to explain why many pharmacists hate their jobs. It has to do with taking a highly motivated, intelligent person, and putting them in a cage, where they are poked with sticks and aggravated, while electronic devices and human voices produce random noise pollution in the background. Oh, and they are also juggling flaming torches and trying not to set anyone on fire.

Pharmacists used to be well respected and had absolute dominion over their pharmacy departments. Somehow, they gradually lost that power and in 2010, at least at Walgreens, the store managers were installed over the pharmacist in charge. Pharmacists are now under the thumb of the store managers, who, although they may have a college degree, have no clue about a pharmacist's job or the weight of responsibility he bears with regard to patient safety. Managers do, however, feel free to pressure the pharmacist to risk his license and livelihood to meet the sales goals set out by the district manager.

Managers and store personnel get breaks and time for lunch, while the pharmacists often cannot get away to eat, drink, or go to the bathroom. As hourly employees, the people running the registers are mandated two 15 minute breaks and a 30 minute lunch during an 8 hour shift. That's right, the high school kid selling you that candy bar gets to rest up from his demanding job, but the pharmacists dispensing your dangerous medication are expected to go up to 14 hours without the same rights to a physical and mental break.

 Put yourself in the pharmacist's shoes on a typical Saturday:

 You leave home at 8:00 am in order to open the pharmacy at 9 am. There is no need to get there earlier to prepare for the day, because you have to wait on the store manager to open the door. You probably worked last night, which in theory allows you to be ahead of the game, since you know what is going on, but mostly really means you are exhausted and defeated before the day even starts.

 You obtain the 3 heavy cash registers from the manager on duty and carry them back to the pharmacy, balancing them on one arm while you struggle to unlock and open the door to the pharmacy department. You will be ringing at all 3 registers today, whether or not you have a technician. You will be expected to ring up anyone who asks, even nonprescription customers who have become frustrated because of the long lines up front. While the technician takes their half hour lunch, and their two fifteen minute breaks, and when they leave for the day, you are on your own.

 You barely get the register drawers in before the drive through bell rings. Despite the sign in the window clearly indicating what time you open, the person in the car decides to sit and wait. Given that you have probably 5 minutes before you open, you try to ignore the drive through and boot up the computer terminals. You make sure you have paper in the printers, check your supply of pens and prescription pads, and go over the notes from the previous day. The drive through bell rings again, which means there is another customer behind the one already waiting. Your stomach begins to churn and your chest and neck muscles tighten.

    You walk over and push the button that raises the garage door in front of the two registers. Already, you can see feet. The effect is of a slow reveal in a movie scene, the kind where the person being revealed is the last person the main character wants to see right now. This person steps forward expectantly and asks for their prescription, which is not here, and which is waiting on your voice mail, because the doctor called it in after you closed last night. When you inform the person that this is not the story of the Elves and the Shoemaker, and their prescription has not been miraculously filled overnight by some unseen hand, they roll their eyes and sigh, and continue to stand at the counter and stare at you.

    You take down the drive through sign and address the customer, who is upset because you waited on the person at the counter when they were here first. You apologize, the first of many apologies you will make today, unless you apologized to the first customer for not performing the impossible, which makes it the second apology you have offered.

The phone begins to ring. If you are a CVS pharmacist, a helpful electronic voice tells you there are X number of calls in the queue. This voice repeats every few minutes in case you forget. A line begins to form at the registers, the drive thru bell is going off, and the phone is ringing. Your technician does not come in until noon, because payroll hours have been cut again.

You page "IC3", if you are at Walgreens, which is super-secret code for "I see 3 customers at the register and I need help". The manager comes back to the pharmacy, and is either condescending, or friendly and helpful. They may know how to help, or they may be clueless and have to ask you what to do. Sometimes the manager is angry with you for interrupting their seemingly more important tasks.

The rest of the day, until you mercifully close the windows at 6 pm and go home, is a soul sucking nightmare. The following may or may not have happened:

A meth head comes in carrying a 2 year old child and asks for Walphed (or the equivalent pseudoephedrine product) in the largest box you have. He makes pleasant chit chat, and tells the child to say "hi" to the "nice lady". When the sale is denied because he has bought pseudoephedrine within the last 7 days, he snarls and calls you a bitch and storms out of the store.

An elderly lady and her husband come in to purchase his new medication. The doctor has chosen the newest thing on the market and it is not available in a generic. Their insurance does not cover it, and it costs $500 per month. The lady begins to cry and tells you he might as well die. You can't contact the doctor until Monday to get a cheaper medication ordered.

A man comes to the counter and throws his inhaler down. He asks how long it will take to fill, and how much it will be. There is no label on the inhaler. You ask him for his name and he is not in the computer. He finally tells you he usually gets it at Walmart for $4, but they are not open yet and he is going out of town. When you say you can't fill it without a transfer from Walmart or a new prescription, he threatens to call corporate and storms out of the store.

A mom comes in with her toddler and hands you a prescription for antibiotics. You can tell they are both exhausted. You tell Mom you will rush the prescription so they can go home. An elderly lady walks up and hands you a plastic bag full of empty prescription bottles, and seems miffed when you tell her it will be 15 minutes. When she persists, you tell her the little boy behind her is very sick and you are going to get his prescription ready first. She softens a bit, and tells the child she knows how he feels, because she has diabetes and heart disease and arthritis. The child stares at her with glazed eyes as she rattles on.

A pain management patient comes in with new prescriptions. His dose has been increased on one of the medications, but he just picked up a large quantity of the same medication in a lower dose two days ago. You remember the prescription was from his general practitioner. You tell him you need to call his pain management doctor to get the okay to go ahead with the prescription. He tells you they are closed today. You tell him you will call Monday. He calls you a bitch and storms out of the store.

These incidents and many more grind away at your psyche, your patience, and your humanity. Even if all the equipment is working properly, you have competent help, and the patients are merciful, the day sucks the life out of you, and you limp out to the parking lot, sit in your car, and wonder how you can ever face one more day of this living hell. You drive home in a fog and hardly know how you got there. You snarl at your spouse or partner, kick the dog, and ignore your kids You head straight for the refrigerator and guzzle down a beer. It tastes fantastic, since you have not eaten or had anything to drink since your morning coffee. Three beers in, your muscles start to loosen and you feel a nice buzz. You could care less about anybody else's day, and you do not want to talk to anybody. If someone calls on the phone, you let it go to voicemail.

You hate yourself, your employer, the people you work with, your patients, and all of humanity. You have sold your soul to the Devil for $100,000 a year, which pretty much disqualifies you from complaining. You work in a clean, safe (except for the robberies, more on that later), air conditioned environment with decent people. What more could you ask for?

Your brother in law, who works in 120 degree heat in a casting plant 7 days a week, does not feel sorry for you. Neither do the people you know who earn considerably less and have to work two jobs to survive. So, you feel sorry for yourself, but refuse to do anything different. You know the pharmacy schools are pumping out new grads and the job market has tightened. You have several colleagues who have disappeared after they complained to management one too many times.

You go to bed after midnight and wake up with a hangover. If anyone should go to church and pray for strength it is you, but unfortunately you work on Sundays, so you snap the Golden Handcuffs on your wrists and head out to face another shitty day.

CHAPTER 7

WORKLOAD AND PATIENT SAFETY

Back in 2014, I decided to contact several investigative reporters to challenge them to go to a busy pharmacy, pose as a customer, and watch and record the chaos that goes on behind the counter. I also contacted Ellen, Oprah, 20/20, CBS, and anybody else I could think of that might be willing to help. I told them that a few hours of watching the train wreck that is modern retail pharmacy was all that they would need to understand the danger inherent in filling prescriptions in such an environment. There was only one response to the over fifty e-mails I sent out. This came from a reporter who wrote "sounds interesting, could you send me more information?" The information was provided to him, and he never responded. This is the e mail I sent out:

I am a retail pharmacist. I am trying to get the word out about the false advertising perpetuated by retail chain pharmacies and the real story of what goes on behind the counter. I would be willing to provide information to combat this huge problem. You will have no problem getting pharmacists to talk if you guarantee they will remain anonymous. We make over $100,000 a year and depend on that income to maintain our lifestyle, but the tradeoff is increasingly a case of diminishing marginal returns. We are all scared for our jobs, and the chains are starting to get rid of us on trivial charges if we show resistance to corporate, or discontent.

1. We often work alone or with technicians who are poorly trained, not suited to the job, have health problems, have stressful or even dangerous home lives, or who have alcohol or substance abuse problems. The chains only pay $10 an hour, which is not enough for a person to live on Some techs work more than one job Some of them are on Medicaid. Some have abusive spouses or partners. The ones with kids often have unreliable or unsafe child care. Most of them have issues that keep them from being fully engaged with their job. In addition to the pressure at home, they are expected to deal with the high stress multitasking environment of retail pharmacy while getting paid about 1/6 of the average pharmacist's pay.

2. Pharmacists are considered management and so we do not get lunch breaks or 15 min breaks. When my blood sugar dips below 70, my thought process is impaired, and I feel "foggy". This is dangerous.

3. I have to run everything when I am without a technician, or when I only have 1 technician. This is most of the time. This includes drive thru and counter, ringing out customers, counseling patients on over the counter products, giving immunizations and health testing, answering the phones, calling insurance companies, and a host of other duties. We are excellent multi-taskers, but there is a breaking point. This is dangerous.

4. Facebook groups "Pharmacists United for Change" and "The Angry Pharmacist Legal Chat" are closed groups dedicated to discussing the problems inherent in modern pharmacy practice.

5. Look at pharmacy blogs like www.pharmaciststeve.com. There are a bunch of links to other pharmacist blogs at this site. These people have been writing for a long time and this should give you a good picture of what is going on

6.Go into a CVS or Walgreens and hang around the pharmacy area where you can observe many of the problems I have pointed out in this email. The chains will not give you permission to film or record because they do not want you to report these abuses.

The trend toward increased services with bare bones staffing is continuing to get worse, and I have not seen anything published about it, except when a pharmacist makes an error, and they parade the poor slob around in front of the media. Even if they say the pharmacist had worked 60 hours in that week with no help, they still try to make it seem as if it is all the pharmacist's fault.

Another angle you should explore is the connection between the big chains and the state boards of pharmacy, and the schools of pharmacy. There is a huge conflict of interest, and no one is representing working pharmacists and helping to keep the public safe from medication errors. For example, Indiana's State Board of Pharmacy President is Bill Cover, who is a Purdue Grad and works for Walgreens. Walgreens CEO Greg Wasson is also a Purdue Grad. I have a nice photo of these two with a bunch of other Purdue grads at the opening of one of the flagship stores they are so proud of.

I hope you seriously consider taking on this project. Whoever does get hold of this will find a wealth of information, discontent among pharmacists, and deception from the big chains and the bean counters who run them. We need someone to get the word out and provide a voice for us and for our patients

Thank you for your consideration,
Kimberly Ankenbruck, RPh

The problem of bare bones staffing and pharmacist workload is nothing new. Payroll is one expense that can be easily controlled, so it is the first expense to be cut when things get tight. Pharmacists understand this, and are able to adapt, to a certain degree. The tipping point for most of us came when the chains started offering immunizations. We handled the flu shots pretty well after we got used to them, working shots into our other daily duties. Then came the shingles shot, and we figured out how to work Zostavax into our workflow. When the chains started offering childhood immunizations and the all the vaccines recommended by the CDC for travelers, the situation became dangerous and unmanageable.

Hard on the heels of the expanded immunization program, came the all day, every day health screenings. Insurance companies started encouraging patients to get dollars added to their HSA accounts by getting an annual health screening and having the appropriate forms filled out. While these health screenings were intended to be performed in the doctor's offices when the patient came in for an annual checkup, corporate decided that the pharmacists could be coerced into using their NPI numbers to bill for health screenings performed in the pharmacy. As a result, we were required to add blood pressure, blood glucose, cholesterol, and body mass screenings to our other responsibilities.

Around this same time, Medicare D patients, and some other insured patients, became eligible for MTM, or Medication Therapy Management. MTM, is a fancy name for having the patient bring in all of their medications for a review and discussion with a pharmacist, and it requires privacy and time to perform properly. Pharmacists generally scheduled these appointments on their time off, since no accommodation was made by the company to support this required task. Unfortunately, since MTM patients who are flagged by their insurance companies to receive this extra service are on multiple medications and have severe health challenges, they often miss these appointments. Understandably, they are not enthused about having to trek to the pharmacy to go over their medications, when they can simply call their doctor or pharmacist from the comfort of their home if they have any questions. MTM is fairly new, and many patients don't understand what it is or how it can help them.

At any rate, although pharmacists develop excellent multitasking skills, there is a limit to what they can keep track of. Multitasking itself is a misnomer, since studies have shown that there is really no such thing. The human brain can only tend to one task at a time. It is estimated that it takes about 30 minutes to resume a task after an interruption. Retail pharmacy is Interruption Central, with a side of antagonism, criticism, danger, fear, and neurochemical overload

The chains cut technician and pharmacist hours at will, and they change their schedules all the time, often with no warning. There are cases where employees have lost their insurance coverage because their hours were cut to under 30 hours a week. In the pharmacy department, this means that the PIC has to take the number of hours of technician help he is allowed to use and spread those hours over the hours the pharmacy is open. He tries to guess when the pharmacy will be busiest, a fool's errand, and schedules his staff accordingly. The pharmacist is responsible for everything that goes on in the pharmacy. Consequently, it behooves him to learn to keep several things in his head at once, to listen with one ear open to what is being said in the background, and to switch from one task to another without dropping the ball. Most of the time this works surprisingly well, although it comes out of the pharmacist's hide. When it doesn't work well, the resultant fallout can range from mildly inconvenient to disastrous.

Floating pharmacists from store to store is another major contributor to medication errors. Often, the only leg the pharmacist has to stand on is that he is familiar with his own store, his own staff, and his own patients. An unfamiliar environment with unfamiliar (or no) help disrupts the thought process from the get go. In addition to the floaters, there are pharmacists who volunteer to pick up shifts at other stores, which means that in addition to being tired from their normal work week, they are also like a fish out of water in an unfamiliar store.

Errors occur in busy, understaffed stores, but, surprisingly, some errors are made on relatively light days, probably because the pharmacist and his staff are more likely to let down their guard. Busy days require laser sharp focus, and an ability to get into "the zone", but light days change the routine and the normal pace of the department.

Error reporting is voluntary and kept in house. At Walgreens, we filled out an online form and reported incidents or errors. They called these "STARS" events. These are supposedly for information purposes only, but it is difficult to report yourself for something that might lead to disciplinary action or firing. Every pharmacist worth his salt will beat himself up over errors and missteps anyway, so filling out the form is simply an in-house record of what occurred, should the need arise to recall the incident later for a patient complaint or a lawsuit.

I once asked if it would be possible to send out an email to our district with the "Top 10 Errors of the Week" or something similar, names and details redacted. My reasoning was simple: if we knew what tripped another pharmacist up, perhaps we could avoid that particular error ourselves. I always say, there are a million ways to screw up, some of which you have never even considered, and forewarned is forearmed. This was met with a lot of head nodding and promises to follow through on the part of the pharmacy DM, and like many of my ideas and the ideas of my colleagues, it was never implemented.

If you want to read more about workload and patient safety, I have included a list of articles in the Appendix. If you have ever worked with the public in a hectic environment, short staffed, unfed and exhausted, while being required to stay pleasant and on top of your game, you can probably skip the extra reading.

At the tippy top of the drug store mountain sits the venerable CEO. Although I have focused primarily on CVS and Walgreens, all of the retail chain pharmacies have similar issues with staffing and workload, as well as non-pharmacist manager oversite of the pharmacy department. The CEOs and their spokespersons are the voice of the company, but they are not speaking the same language as the pharmacists in their employ, nor does anything coming out of their mouths resemble what is being said by the pharmacists, the other store employees, or the customers. Although some of the executives are pharmacists, one gets the impression that they are only too happy to have used their education to climb out from the pits of hell and become Top Dog over the minions who do their bidding at store level. All of them have thrown the rest of us under the big fat corporate bus and backed up and over us a few times for good measure.

Greg Wasson is a pharmacist and the former CEO of Walgreens. He "retired" at 56, jumping ship with his Golden Parachute after the Walgreens-Boots Alliance merger. As I have already mentioned, immunizations, health screenings, and MTMs were instituted under his leadership. He was also at the helm for the "Rewiring for Growth" campaign. "Rewiring for Growth" jacked around a lot of long time, loyal employees, moving them to other stores, adding more duties for the same salary or cutting salaries, cutting hours for support staff, and generally shaking up the whole organization with the intent of keeping everybody off balance and afraid. Fear is a great motivator, and the Big Boys had the Wag Slaves scrambling to accommodate their demands under Wasson's directives.

  After the merger, Wasson abruptly handed off the company to Stefano Pessina, an Italian born nuclear engineer and drug wholesaler. who was formerly executive chairman of Alliance Boots, and is now acting CEO of Walgreens Boots Alliance. His life partner of over 30 years, Ornella Barra, is a qualified pharmacist and Co-Chief Operating Officer of the company. Her website, ornellabarra.com, shows just how dedicated and in touch she remains with the profession of pharmacy. Photos of Barra scroll across the top of the page, captioned with profound and insightful quotes like this one: "I love pharmacy. It brings healthcare to communities."

  Larry Merlo is the CEO of CVS Health. He is a 1978 graduate of the University of Pittsburgh School of pharmacy. In 2014, he announced that CVS would no longer sell tobacco products in its stores. He also expanded the company's line of "Minute Clinics, projecting an increase from 800 to 1500 locations by 2017. In 2015, it was announced that Merlo had the highest

CEO-to-average-employee-pay-ratio of any American company, according to Forbes Magazine. During his tenure, CVS has been criticized for understaffing, not allowing pharmacy staff to take breaks, and underfunding critical aspects of daily operations. (Fortune 2015) (Glassdoor 2011) (Tribune 2016)

George Riedl was the senior vice president of Walmart health and wellness from 2015 to March 2018. He is a pharmacist, as is his wife, Melanie, and nine of his family members. Mr. Riedl is licensed as a pharmacist in the state of Illinois, but his bio indicates that he has not spent much time behind the bench. He has mainly worked as a buyer in various positions, including a 27- year stint as a buyer for Walgreens. The pharmacists who work in his stores do not seem to be enamored with the way the pharmacy department was run under his leadership. According to a former pharmacist who posted on Indeed.com in 2015:

"Not recommended. Work life balance, job security, and advancement is terrible here. Management tends to work against you rather than with you. They expect so much while giving so little, in terms of a supporting staff. You're expected to be available for them 24 hours a day without being paid that way." (Indeed.com 2015)

Rite Aid corporation is currently the third largest pharmacy chain, behind CVS and Walgreens. It became the third largest drug store chain by acquiring Gray Drug and Read's Drug Store (1987), Peoples Drugs (1989), Hook's Drug Stores (from Revco, 1994), Thrifty PayLess (1996), Harco, Inc. and K&B Inc. (late 1990's), and EnvisionRx (PBM, 2015). Rite Aid's Senior Vice President of Pharmacy Services, is a graduate of the Quinlan School of Business, Loyola University, Chicago. Here is his profile on Linked In. Sounds like a man who has his finger on the pulse of the pharmacy profession to me.

"Seasoned senior technology executive with 27 years of program and project management experience in the financial services industry. A proven turnaround specialist and change agent with history of successfully restructuring departments and programs. Chris is a collaborative business partner and process-oriented leader, known for building and empowering highly motivated cross-functional teams which have consistently delivered results and optimized technology investments." (Linkedin 2017)

Glassdoor and Indeed.com have numerous online testimonials from pharmacists and technicians who work for CVS, Walgreens, and Walmart. They attest to the usual shortcomings in the pharmacy workplace, including lack of adequate support staff, overwork, lack of security, and dangerous, chaotic conditions affecting patient safety and employee health.

In 2011, Walmart decided to promise that up to 3 prescriptions would be filled within 15 minutes, or the customer would receive a $5 gift card. This bit of lunacy probably added up to quite a few $5 windfalls for customers, who were unaware or didn't care that rushing the pharmacist is never a good idea. Even Domino's Pizza used to have a 30 -minute guarantee for pizza, but they dropped the promotion after several of their drivers had car accidents while rushing to make the deadline for delivery.

While the chains nickel and dime their employees to death, squeezing every bit of profit they can from the poor suckers who work for them, they seem to have no problem passing out $25 gift cards to any customer who doesn't get their way, or who utters so much as a peep about "poor service" or "employee attitude". They happily pay millions of dollars in fines, settlements, and judgements that are the result of their poor decisions, while denying any wrong doing on their part. The perception that prescriptions can be cranked out in 15 minutes or less, safely, accurately, and without fail, leads us to our next subject: the adversarial relationship between pharmacists and customers (formerly referred to as patients).

But, before we go there, let us take a segue into a fantasy near and dear to my heart, one that I have replayed over and over, with different variations on the theme, but always with the aim of making these rich pimps experience a day from hell similar to the ones their pharmacists endure, day after day, year after year.

CHAPTER 8

A PHARMACIST'S FANTASY

"Back to you, Gary!"

She laughed, punchy and weary, but glad to be on the last leg of her journey. She started the truck and pulled out onto the county road. In minutes, she was at the old gas station. She checked her phone screen. Gary was still hanging in the parachute harness with his head hanging down, chin resting on his chest. He was snoring.

"Hello, Mr. Williams" Krista said thru the voice changer.

Gary jumped.

"I have questions. You will answer them. Or else." She stifled a snicker at her imitation of the great Man Bat.

"God dammit, get me down from here, you son of a bitch!" Gary was furious, practically foaming at the mouth.

"What's the matter, Mr. Williams, are you tired, hungry, and on your last nerve? Welcome to the world you created for your pharmacists!"

Gary lurched around and cursed for a few minutes, but he was clearly exhausted. Krista looked at her watch. Gary's captivity was heading into its 15th hour.

"Oopsy daisy, looks like you had to work over! Well, you're a professional, you're expected to do what it takes to accommodate the patients, because their Health and Happiness is Our Number One Priority, right Gare?"

More lurching and cursing from the captive CEO ensued. He was clearly near the end of his rope. Krista was getting tired herself, and she had more than made her point. Maybe she should have let Karma take care of this bastard, but the problem with Karma was it took a long time and you usually never found out about the results.

Krista fired up the remote for the shock collar. She sent Williams a test shock.

"Fuck! God damn it!" Gary swung around violently, kicking his feet and waving his arms around. "Jesus Christ, I'll fucking kill you!"

"I doubt it, Gary. Now, I am going to ask you a series of questions. If you answer them incorrectly or do not know the answer, you will get a shock. If you answer correctly, you get nothing, just like the pharmacists you employ get when they provide their knowledge for free, all day, every day."

"Question number one. Your diabetic patient comes in stating that her blood sugar has been running around 300 in the morning when she tests. How should she adjust her insulin regimen so her sugars don't run so high in the morning?"

"Shit, I don't know, I haven't practiced in years, you know that, asshole. I don't give a damn."

"That is incorrect." Krista administered a shock. Gary cursed and flailed.

"Question number two. What would you recommend for a 7 year old child who is running a fever, with an inner ear infection, swimmers ear, and sinus drainage?"

Gary clenched his jaw and stared straight ahead.

"Gee, you sure seemed to know a lot about our job when you were calling the shots from your castle of doom, Gare, what's wrong, Cat Woman got your tongue? She does that, it's just her way." Shock administered.

"Question number three."

"How many fucking questions are you going to ask me?"

"Oh, you never know. Day to day it could be hundreds, and some have nothing to do with pharmacy. Should I ask you where the colored toothpicks are? 'Cause I'm guessing you don't know." Shock administered.

Krista turned off the voice changer and let Gary dangle for a while. Then, she shocked him one more time, just for good measure, before turning off the remote. She was on her last legs and wanted to wrap up this caper before she got too tired and started making stupid mistakes. She retrieved the dart gun from her bag and loaded a ketamine cartridge into the chamber. She raised the gun to her shoulder and stuck the barrel through a small hole she had cut in the drywall. Gary was facing the side wall, his head hanging down again. This shot was going to be a little more difficult due to the dog collar. But, on the other hand, there was plenty of light, and she didn't need to worry about her prey going anywhere. She carefully shined the red laser dot onto the white skin of Gary's neck.

"Goodnight, sweet prince!"

Gary slumped in his harness. Krista put the dart gun back in her duffle bag and gathered the rest of her gear. She opened the side passenger door and tossed the bag into the seat. Then she went around and opened the tailgate, and slid a steel ramp into place. She went back inside the building to retrieve Gary. She lowered him down slowly, and unhooked him from the pulley system, letting his body fall in a heap on the floor. She opened the gray metal door and propped it open with a piece of wood. Then she dragged Gary across the gravel to the back of the Escalade. She pulled him part way up the ramp, propping his body on the incline until she could scramble around and through the truck and grab his harness before he slid back down.

"Good God, I starved the asshole, and I think he's gained 10 pounds!"

Krista grunted and yanked until Gary's feet were clear of the back door. She slid out via the side door and went around to the back of the SUV to close the lift gate.

"Okay, I think that's it. Well, Gare, it's time to release you from your human bondage. Ashes to ashes, dust to dust. Asses to asses, busts to busts. Assholes to strip malls, left in the dust."

Krista drove the thirty miles to the little strip mall she had seen on her way to and from the gas station. Of all the possible drop off points she had passed in her travels, this one seemed to be the best option. A Save A Lot grocery store anchored the location, along with a Dollar General and a Big Lots. The parking lot was poorly lit, and the stores sat back from the road, so it was hard to see anything if you were just driving by. Since the stores opened at 9 am, Krista figured Gary wouldn't be out here too long before someone came in to open one of the businesses.

She shut the vehicle off and circled around to the back, opening the lift gate with the button on her key fob. She pulled the ramp into place and grasped both of Gary's ankles, pulling him to the top of the ramp and sliding him part way down. She unbuckled the parachute harness and slid the straps down his body until she had extricated him from the contraption. Then, she got behind him and grabbed him in a bear hug, working him off the ramp and onto the ground. She dragged him to the sidewalk in front of the grocery store. She got a blanket and pillow from the Escalade and ran back to cover him with the blanket and prop his head on the pillow. She had considered pouring a few shots of whisky on him and propping the bottle in his hands so he would look like an old vagrant who had passed out from too much Wild Turkey, but he looked so pathetic lying there she figured she would spare him that indignity.

"Well, Mr. Williams, it has been a pleasure doing business with you."

She resisted the urge to give him one last swift kick before taking her leave. She laughed and shook her head at her nuttiness.

"Girl, you have done lost it, that's all I have to say" she said as she removed her gloves and wiped her hands on her pants, and hoisted herself up into the Escalade for the long drive home.

CHAPTER 9

THE CUSTOMER IS ALWAYS RIGHT

Sometimes, customers, for I hesitate to call them patients any more, are their own worst enemies, and their expectations, actions and abuse are not only tolerated but often rewarded with $25 gift cards. This monster has been created by the corporations. The customer is always right has done much to degrade the business of retail, and pharmacy is no exception.

The day patients became customers was a black day for us all. Don't get me wrong, pharmacy has always been a service profession and we take that very seriously. However, by virtue of our degree in Pharmacy and our license in the state in which we practice, we are considered drug experts and as such, we are responsible for making sure our patients are not harmed.

Pharmacists were respected, not so very long ago. There was a time that if a patient decided they didn't want to listen to their healthcare providers, or if they decided to try and coerce their doctor or pharmacist into acting against their principles or their better judgement, particularly if they used abusive language or became violent, they were told to kindly take their business elsewhere It seems like the weather began to shift when some retailers loosened their returned goods policies and began taking back products without a receipt. I don't know when this happened, exactly, but looking back, I really think this was the beginning.

I have taken advantage of the more lenient policies born of increased competition, just like everybody else. I can't always find my receipt, I have kept items too long before returning them, I have forgotten where I bought an item and tried to return it at the wrong store. I assume retailers have seen an increase in sales by bending over backwards to accommodate customers and give them what they want. Otherwise, there would be no incentive to allow returns any time, with no receipt, and no questions asked. Similarly, there would be no reason to offer free shipping both ways, allow the use of coupons and vouchers in addition to the sale price, or to issue "rewards" to be used toward the customer's next purchase. Pharmacy is different, or it should be.

While I definitely want to be in charge of my own healthcare decisions, and I expect to be given accurate advice regarding the risks and benefits of any treatment recommended by my healthcare providers, I realize I do not have the knowledge or experience to figure out what my best course of action should be. That is why I hire an expert. If I don't like what the expert has to say, or if I can't establish a workable patient/provider relationship with the individual practitioner, or if I can't afford the services of this professional, I go elsewhere. Eventually, I will get a consensus and decide on a treatment plan, based on the options I have been offered.

Once I select a practitioner based on qualities I value, like competence, dependability, follow through, communication, honesty, integrity, clarity, empathy, and courtesy, I put myself in their hands. I assume this professional has my best interests at heart and is going to do everything in their power to help me. I rarely complain about having to wait past my appointment time in my doctor's office. I assume he is busy with his other patients, and that he will give the same kind attention to me when it is my turn. I schedule my appointment first thing in the morning to try and avoid the snowball effect that happens when appointments start to overlap. If I have a long wait every time I have an appointment, I consider whether this doctor's expertise is worth waiting for. If it is, I may state my opinion to the receptionist or nurse, but I do not storm back to the treatment room and give him both barrels about having to wait. Somehow, I do not think this would be in my best interest.

  In contrast, some patients that we encounter in the pharmacy treat us as if we are no more than burger flippers, preparing patties instead of poison. While most people understand that it would be ludicrous to walk into any other professional's office without an appointment and expect to be served immediately by the practitioner himself, they have been taught by the chains that this is perfectly acceptable behavior when dealing with pharmacists. Being the "most accessible healthcare professionals" is a two-edged sword. The title used to be a source of pride, indicating that we were friendlier, less intimidating, more down to earth. Now, it means that we are standing in the eye of a hurricane and expected to be all things to all people without the resources to do our jobs properly.

People who wait patiently for their tall mocha latte at Starbuck's, and understand that it takes time to create their favorite specialty drink, are often the same people who get upset when they have to wait more than 15 minutes for a prescription. Customers who drop off their prescriptions and offer to come back later, call their refills a few days ahead of time, bring in their new insurance card, understand when a medication is out of stock and must be ordered, and patiently wait for the pharmacist to acknowledge them and prepare their order, are few and far between. In fact, they are so rare that when we encounter one of these individuals, we are likely to get tears in our eyes and practically kiss their feet with gratitude.

The chains have set you and I up to have an adversarial relationship. Pharmacists are now the enemy, because we look like bumbling buffoons as we juggle too many tasks with too few resources. We have to wear too many hats.

Does your doctor greet you at the receptionist's desk, process your insurance, collect your copay, answer the office phones personally by the third ring, gather the materials needed for your exam, clean the room after your exam, order supplies and put them away, and generally run the whole office by himself? Of course not. Pharmacists have allowed the chains to take over our profession, and this is the unfortunate result. The reason pharmacy has gone from the most trusted profession to an all-out war of wills is part of the larger problem of putting healthcare in the hands of corporations.

Pharmacists are not off the hook for the relationship we have with the public, far from it. Pharmacists who are smart asses, who make snide remarks, demean patients, spend their time scrolling through messages on their cell phone or yacking with the techs instead of working, are loathed by other pharmacists and techs as well as by patients. The best of us have bad days.

I have "lost it" with patients and other employees, I have been guilty of talking and laughing and keeping patients waiting, and I have been grumpy, surly, and sarcastic. I kick myself when I indulge in these behaviors, but that does not excuse them. For me, these slip ups are born of frustration, both with the system and with the lack of understanding and the impatience of the public. I want to do a good job and keep my patients safe. Many of these lapses in professionalism are a result of too many hours without a break or food or a bathroom break. Over the years, I have found that when my blood sugar goes below 70, I get "hangry". Unfortunately, I do not have the option of sitting down to a meal, and every minute I spend eating or trying to eat takes away from the time I could be using to fill prescriptions and get myself out of the weeds.

In the heat of battle, when somebody pushes one of my buttons, I sometimes respond inappropriately. Like the dung beetle who pushes his ball of poop up an incline, only to have it roll over him and back down the hill, the Sisyphean reality of retail pharmacy practice feels like so much "pounding sand down a rat hole" with no end or relief in sight.

CHAPTER 10

STATE BOARDS OF PHARMACY

One subject that has been too rarely addressed is the responsibility of the state boards of pharmacy, and the attorney general who oversees them, to protect the public. While pharmacists are held to the strictest standards of conduct and professional ethics, the companies they work for seem to get a free pass from the officials who have been given the power, by law, to regulate the practice of pharmacy. The current staffing and excessive workloads continue, despite repeated complaints from pharmacists and patients alike. There does not seem to be any accountability when these government officials fail to follow through on their responsibilities, but they are all too willing to bring the hammer down on individual pharmacists and reprimand them if they make an error in judgement or harm a patient. The mission statements of the state boards of pharmacy clearly state that they are responsible for the safety of patients. Consider the following examples:

MISSOURI BOARD OF PHARMACY

It is the mission of the Board of Pharmacy and the Division of Professional Registration to serve and protect the public by providing an accessible, responsible and accountable regulatory system that protects the public from incompetency, misconduct, gross negligence, fraud, misrepresentation or dishonesty, licenses only "qualified" professionals by examination and evaluation of minimum competency, and enforces standards by implementing legislation and administrative rules.

NORTH CAROLINA BOARD OF PHARMACY

The North Carolina Board of Pharmacy's mission is to protect the public health, safety and welfare in pharmaceutical matters. The Board sets standards for academic and practical experience programs prior to licensure, issues permits to operate pharmacies and DME facilities, and annually renews licenses, permits and registrations.

OKLAHOMA BOARD OF PHARMACY

The Mission of the Oklahoma State Board of Pharmacy is to protect the health, safety, and welfare of the citizens of Oklahoma by regulating and enforcing the laws regarding the practice of pharmacy and the manufacturing, sale, distribution and storage of drugs, medicines, chemicals and poisons.

INDIANA BOARD OF PHARMACY

The practice of pharmacy is declared to be a professional occupation in the state of Indiana, affecting the public health, safety, and welfare and must be subject to regulation and control in the public interest by the board of pharmacy. It is further declared to be a matter of public interest and concern that the practice of pharmacy merit and receive the confidence of the public and that only qualified persons be permitted to practice pharmacy in the state of Indiana In addition, the Board of Pharmacy is to: "establish requirements and tests to determine the moral, physical, intellectual, educational, scientific, technical, and professional qualifications for applicants for pharmacists' license."

Despite these high- minded statements, state boards of pharmacy have failed to uphold these standards when dealing with the powerful chain drug stores like Walgreens and CVS. They have abdicated their responsibility in this regard, choosing instead to turn a blind eye to what the chains are doing, while emphatically enforcing the responsibilities of the individual pharmacist to stand firm in his professional convictions in the face of corporate pressure to perform, and threats of job loss. This duty to uphold the law falls under the dreaded phrase "use your professional judgement". While this statement may seem to offer support for the pharmacists' judgement, it in fact provides a loophole that has allowed employers to hold pharmacists accountable for adverse consequences while mandating metrics and policies that are in direct opposition to the pharmacist's duties.

This "head in the sand" behavior is further bolstered by the fact that many of the state board members are employed by chain stores, and several of them have been caught using their power as board members to advance the agenda of the companies they work for. An ABC news report from December 30, 2008 references an investigation by USA Today entitled "Chain Pharmacies Run Deep in Boards of Pharmacy" which brings to light the number of retail chain pharmacists represented on the state boards of pharmacy. The report cites a quote attributed to Daniel Hussar, a pharmacy professor at Philadelphia's University of the Sciences and editor of the Pharmacist Activist newsletter:

"The chains aggressively seek as much representation on the boards as they possibly can". (TODAY 2008)

Although the chains vigorously deny the existence of any conflict of interest, insisting that their employees on the State Boards are careful to recuse themselves when matters before the Board are of concern to their employers, the fact remains that there are multiple instances in which this is just not true. In one of the more blatant examples of this abuse of power, William J Cover, who in 2011 was both president of the Indiana Board of Pharmacy and Manager of Pharmacy Affairs for Walgreens, used his position on the Board to influence voting in favor of the Well at Walgreens store model being considered by the company. The model, which features the pharmacist out in front of the pharmacy with a computer and a phone, and the technicians in back filling prescriptions, has been widely criticized because of patient privacy concerns and the possibility of increased errors. The traditional pharmacy model requires direct and personal supervision of pharmacy technicians by the pharmacist, rather than verification of prescriptions via a remote screen. The screen is hidden from view in the traditional model, but the Well at Walgreens model leaves the screen clearly visible to other patients and shoppers, especially if the pharmacist is called away. Despite these concerns, and pushback by two citizen groups, Common Cause Indiana, and Change to Win, the Well at Walgreens model was pushed through. Indiana regulations were modified in 2013 to allow certain types of remote supervision, thus sanctioning the final piece required to go ahead with the project. (John Russel 2014)

The chains exert pressure via their state board members any time they want a change that benefits their business. Each state has a law that mandates how many technicians can be under the direct supervision of one pharmacist. According to Jim "Goose" Rawlings, a pharmacist in Lafayette, Indiana, who has a friend on the Indiana Board of Pharmacy with no retail pharmacy connections:

"The BOP has 7 members, but by law only 1 has to be a hospital pharmacist, and 1 is a consumer member with no connection to pharmacy. I'm sure the other 5 are retail people. My friend tells me the major chains are always trying to get the board to relax rules so they can cut staff. Indiana has a law that a pharmacist can only supervise 4 technicians at one time. The chains try to get this relaxed so they can add more technicians without adding pharmacist overlap." (Drug Topics 2011)

Pharmacists have regaled board members for years, trying to get them to do their jobs and take control of the situation in retail pharmacies. Instead of helping, they have colluded with the chains, quietly sneaking in new legislation, such as Senate Bill 0407, passed March 9, 2012, which increased the number of pharmacy technicians that may be supervised by one pharmacist from 4 to 6 in Indiana. Every pharmacist knows that it is hard enough to keep track of what 4 technicians are doing, let alone 6. Keep in mind that some or all of the 6 may be technicians in training, or new employees, which is a whole other area of concern. (Indiana General Assembly Archive). Incidentally, Indiana and Idaho currently have the highest technician to pharmacist ratio at 6:1. For a run down on the ratio in other states, see the article entitled "Pharmacy Technician Regulation" in Pharmacy Times (Pharmacy Times 2016)

Some State Boards have begun to wake up and address the problems in the pharmacist workplace. A letter written by Steven F. Anderson Rph., a member of the Washington State Quality Assurance Commission, includes a sampling of rules that some of the state boards of pharmacy have implemented relating to staffing, workload, performance metrics and quotas, meals and breaks, quality control, space for clinical services, transfer incentives, and accountability. (Washington State Quality Assurance Commission 2015) Still, the standard answer given by the majority of the state boards when challenged about why they refuse to address problems like pharmacist work load, staffing, lack of breaks and lunch, and the impact these conditions have on patient safety, is *"We are not in the business of telling employers what to do."*

If this is the case, what are they here for? And who, then, is ultimately responsible for policing these corporations when they put the public in danger? By default, the individual pharmacist is expected to uphold the laws and ethics of the profession against the onslaught of the corporate juggernaut, despite the fact that an entire agency charged with this very responsibility refuses to act in the interest of public safety.

CHAPTER 11

THE GOVERNMENT

I have already mentioned that the attorneys general of the states are responsible for overseeing the boards of pharmacy, but they have failed to act in this regard, choosing instead to go after the low hanging fruit that is easily plucked. It is much easier to blame individual healthcare professionals and hold them up as an example, rather than take on a whole system that is corrupt and rife with conflicts of interest and abuses of power on a grand scale. If the state boards of pharmacy and the attorneys general are not going to do their jobs, then perhaps other state and federal government officials should step in. Surely, they have not been influenced by contributions from big corporations. Yeah, right. And stop calling me Shirley.

Anyway, as you know, the government is currently engaged in fiddling around with healthcare, playing Game of Thrones with our lives, and God knows what they really know or what, if any, advice they are getting from people who actually work at the ground level in healthcare. If they are refusing to listen to the professionals who do know what is going on, while accepting campaign donations from Big Pharma, Big Chain Pharmacy, Big Hospital, Big Insurance, and Big Stockholders, you can guess who has the biggest influence on their decisions. (Federal Election Commission 2017) (PAC 2017)

Since doctors, nurses, pharmacists, and all the other healthcare personnel who have been mostly swallowed up in the Great Medical Machine don't have Big Money, they have no voice. Similarly, the patients sitting at the bottom of this shit storm are easily disregarded. After all, they need medication. How and when they get it, how much it costs, and what it does or doesn't do for them is irrelevant to the Top Dogs of Medical Mania, as long as they can keep the money rolling in, and maintain their high prestige corporate and government jobs with all the attendant perks.

An article on the New Yorker website (newyorker.com) by Jeffrey Frank, dated January 17, 2017 and entitled "On Health Care, We'll Have What Congress is Having" gives a pretty clear description of the history of the fight for universal health care. (Frank 2017). What follows is a description of the insurance plan enjoyed by Congress before the Affordable Care Act was passed in 2010.

"The F.E.H.B.P., as it's known, was started in 1959, a few years before Medicare, and was meant to cover some nine million government employees—civil-service workers, the courts, the Post Office, members of Congress, and more. It wasn't a single plan but, rather, as a Times story put it, "a supermarket offering 300 private health plans." (Even the right-leaning Heritage Foundation called it "a showcase of consumer choice and free-market competition.") One may get a sense of its scope and inclusiveness—its supermarket-ness—in the way that the Office of

Personnel Management, which administers the program, explains it to federal employees. Much of the program—for instance, the idea that no one can be refused, or charged more, for a preexisting condition, or that dependents under twenty-six are covered—will sound familiar to anyone conversant with the most attractive parts of the Affordable Care Act."

After the Affordable Care Act was passed in 2010, government officials became ineligible for F.E.H.B.P. For all its flaws, bumbled launch, and absence of Republican support, the A.C.A. has provided health insurance to some twenty million Americans who didn't have it before. Republicans have been venomously eager to dismantle it ever since. Late last week, the Senate took a big step in that direction by passing a budget "blueprint" that will make it easy for Congress, controlled by Republicans, to repeal the act.

If it's sometimes hard to understand what makes Republican legislators so angry, here is a theory: their fury may not stem from some ungraspable principle, or hatred of President Obama's historic victory (or of Obama himself), but, rather, from something personal, and selfish. Under the A.C.A., members of Congress, and congressional staff, among other Capitol Hill employees, were no longer eligible for the F.E.H.B.P. In the chilly language of government directives, the Office of Personnel Management Web site said that "Section 1312 of the Affordable Care Act requires that Members of Congress and their official staff obtain coverage by health plans created under the Affordable Care Act or coverage offered via an Affordable Insurance Exchange.

Under the Affordable Care Act, members of the U.S. House of Representatives, the Senate, and their office staffs who want employer coverage generally have to buy it on the health insurance exchange. Before the ACA passed in 2010, they were eligible to be covered under the Federal Employees Health Benefits Program. (People working for congressional committees who are not on a member's office staff may still be covered under F.E.H.B.)." (Andrews 2017) **(Frank 2017) (Frank 2017) (Frank 2017)**

While the state boards of pharmacy deserve their share of the blame for refusing to address pharmacists' working conditions, the government often intentionally stands in the way of even the simplest of requests, like a 30 -minute uninterrupted meal break for pharmacists.

In response to the Chicago Tribune articles previously cited, regarding the lack of diligence displayed by pharmacists in catching serious drug interactions, State Rep. Mary Flowers, D-Chicago, sponsored legislation that would restrict the hours pharmacists can work each day, limit the number of prescriptions they can fill each hour, require break time during their shifts, and provide whistleblower protection if they expose safety problems (Zbigniew Bzdak/Chicago Tribune).

Rep. Flowers also addressed the need for whistleblower protection in her proposed bill.

"They have to add whistleblower, because right now they're all afraid to speak" Flowers said, saying the pharmacists face an *"amazing"* fear of retaliation.

Illinois Governor Bruce Rauner told the Chicago Tribune that he was worried that limits on pharmacist hours and other restrictions could *"raise up costs and don't really increase safety"*. What Governor Rauner fails to realize is that pharmacists have been required to counsel on every prescription since the Omnibus Budget Reconciliation Act of 1990. OBRA-90 was enacted by the federal government in an attempt to save money by mandating pharmacists to counsel, perform prospective drug utilization reviews (ProDur) to look for drug interactions and other problems, and to conform to certain record keeping mandates. While OBRA-90 was meant to improve medication outcomes for Medicaid patients, the states decided to include all patients in the mandate rather than setting up two sets of standards, one for Medicaid patients and one for non-Medicaid patients.

The pro-business pharmacy lobby started attacking the bill before Rep. Flowers could even set a date for hearings. Rob Karr, president of the Illinois Retail Merchants Association, said his group will be *"pursuing active opposition"*, and that the governor's suggestions for enhancing safety through legislation requiring pharmacists to counsel patients with the first prescription, or when prescriptions change, are improvement enough (Chicago Tribune 2017).

This vehement opposition and idiotic disregard of the facts is at the root of the frustration experienced by everyone who works in the healthcare field. If we can't even get as far as letting pharmacists eat an uninterrupted lunch, a basic human need enjoyed by every other worker, what hope do we have of making any significant changes in how our practice is run by the corporations?

Once again, the elephant in the living room has been ignored. Laws and mandates mean nothing when corporations are not required to provide the staffing required to support these mandates. We used to counsel before we lost control of our profession. We are dying to counsel now. Too bad the onus has once again been placed on the individual pharmacist to kill themselves to make an unworkable and untenable situation work. God forbid the government take on the Big Chain Boys. What this says about government officials and their priorities and loyalties is telling. I believe we would be better off voting every single one of them out of office and replacing them, but only after corporations (who are now considered "citizens" for the purposes of campaign contributions) and lobbyists are prohibited from making campaign contributions. In fact, I would go as far as to throw all the lobbyists out of Washington and allow individuals and groups of citizens to speak directly to Congress and the President through any means they deem appropriate.

The political/corporate rat king lives off the rest of us, their tails intertwined, with so many conflicts of interest that issues important to our well-being and survival are never addressed, and we remain stuck with the status quo (Wikipedia 2017)

FIGURE 1 THE POLITICAL AND CORPORATE RAT KING (RAT-KING 1993)

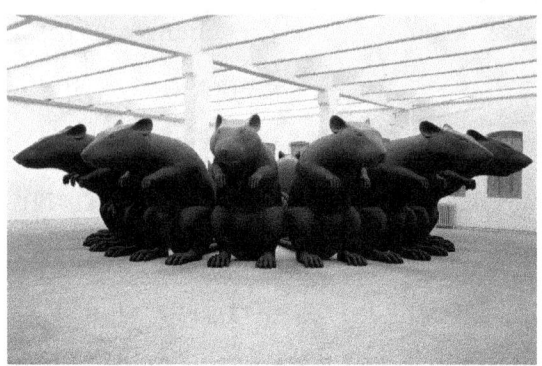

CHAPTER 12
SCHOOLS OF PHARMACY

The schools of pharmacy have a conflict of interest when it comes to teaching students what really goes on in the pharmacy, vs. what they wish was going on. After all, they accept money from the pharmacy chains and pharmaceutical companies. If they want students to learn what is possible in a pharmacy utopia, perhaps they should offer courses on how to engage with the powers that be to effect change in the profession. Instead, they ignore the sad fact that they themselves are afraid to speak up to the corporations for fear of losing funding or sources of employment for their graduates.

The Pharmacy Schools are in the pockets of Walgreens and CVS, who make large donations and sponsor "Career Days", with the expectation that the schools will continue to crank out graduates who have been fed lies about what a pharmacist actually does, saddling these young professionals with $250,000 in student loans and a strong incentive to do whatever their bosses tell them to do to keep their jobs.

Greg Wasson, the CEO of Walgreens before he "retired" at 56, (American Journal of Pharmaceutical Education 2007) following the merger with Boots Alliance, is himself a 1981 graduate of the Purdue School of Pharmacy. Purdue has showered Wasson with awards while ignoring the fact that he was at the helm when Walgreens began descent into madness, taking the whole profession and its pharmacists along for the ride. (The Purdue Pharmacist 2012)

Does corporate giving influence schools of pharmacy and their pharmacy graduates? A study published in the Journal of Pharmaceutical Education in 2007 says it does. Administrative officials from 11 colleges and schools of pharmacy in the United States were surveyed, and the results indicated that about half of the respondents agreed that accepting corporate gifts could lead to real or potential problems with regard to conflicts of interest. 61% thought that corporate gifts had an influence on students.

What really steams pharmacy graduates, including those from my generation (class of 1984, Purdue University School of Pharmacy) is the plain and simple fact that the schools lied to us. They didn't tell us that there were very few positions out there for pharmacists to use their knowledge in a clinical setting. The majority of us would end up slaves to the mechanics of transferring pills and liquids from big containers to smaller containers, typing and sticking labels on said containers, billing for the medication, and trying to relate what we considered important information to a hostile creature standing before us who just wants to go home.

Personally, I don't know why I wasted my time taking organic chemistry, biochemistry, pharmacology, pharmacokinetics, and medicinal chemistry. I would have been better off taking courses like the Psychology of the Angry Customer, Assertiveness for Dummies, Speed Filling for the Modern Pharmacist, How to Multitask Without Killing Someone, How to Fix Printers and other Office Equipment, How to Handle the Narcissist, and How to Keep from Taking it Personally When Someone Screams in Your Face.

Some pharmacists would argue that I if I had applied myself and developed myself professionally, I would have been able to work in a clinical position and have a more fulfilling career. I would argue that I am one of the hard -working staff pharmacists who did the shit work so a lucky few could wear a clean lab coat, attend meetings and seminars, hob nob with doctors and other health care professionals, and eat lunch and use the bathroom like normal human beings.

Our parents are also complicit in this web of lies. They taught us that hard work, integrity, honesty, character, and ability were the keys to a successful career, when, in reality, the modern keys to success are ass kissing, schmoozing, networking and "team building", in addition to lying, cheating, and throwing other people under the bus. In other words, it's not the smart, capable bird, or even the early bird, that gets the worm. It's the bird with the dazzling beak, the fancy plumage, and the pretty song who knows how to kick the other birds out of the nest.

FIGURE 2 WALGREENS EXECS WITH PURDUE PHARMACY ALUMS

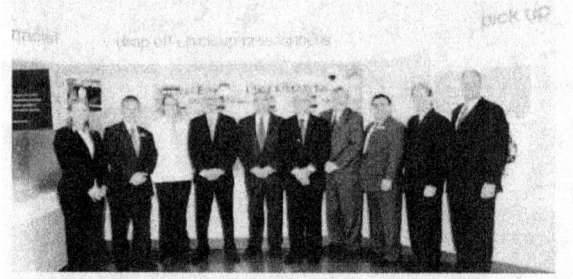

Walgreens representatives and Purdue Pharmacy alumni gather at the dedication in Indianapolis (L. to R) Kelly Baranko, Mark Smosna (BS 1999), Jill Biss (PharmD 2010), Greg Wasson (BS 1981), Ron Rosich (BS 1981), Marvin Richardson (BS 1980), Senior Associate Dean Holly Mason, Stevan Mizimakoski (BS 1999), Bill Cover (BS 1989), and David Lovejoy (BS 1982)

FIGURE 3 WALGREENS GIVES CHECK TO PURDUE SCHOOL OF PHARMACY

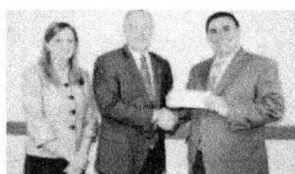

Walgreens representatives Erin Meeker, Pharmacy Campus Relations Manager, and **Stevan Mizimakoski** (BS 1999), Pharmacy Supervisor, present a check to Dean Craig Svensson on February 2, 2012 to continue their support of pharmacy scholarships and Multicultural Programs.

CHAPTER 13

PROFESSIONAL ORGANIZATIONS

Pharmacy's professional organizations are lame ducks, touting the great opportunities for pharmacists, like providing immunizations, performing health screenings, and billing for medication management services, while ignoring the fact that these duties are supposed to be carried out at the same time prescriptions are being filled, phones answered, customers rung up, patients counseled, and all the other legal and ethical tasks required of a pharmacist.

The NABP, AACP, ASHP, ASCP, ACCP, CPNP, and a host of other well initialed groups constantly harangue pharmacists about advancing the profession through increasing clinical functions, while their colleagues in the trenches just try to get through another day without hurting or killing someone. The fact that not one of these organizations has had the wherewithal to address the problems of insufficient staffing and workload in the pharmacy is telling.

In my state, the IPA, or Indiana Pharmacists Alliance, states on its website (indianapharmacists.org) that its office in Indianapolis has "a small staff dedicated to advancing pharmacy in Indiana". Good luck with that. Most of the pharmacists I know would much rather vent their frustrations to their colleagues over an IPA at their local watering hole than support one more lame organization that does nothing to address the obvious problems with their working conditions while seeking to add even more tasks that their employers can hire them out for to extract more money from the unsuspecting public. I filed my recent flyer from them in the circular file without even reading it.

As the profession they represent burns to the ground, the state and local pharmacist organizations spend their time wondering why their membership numbers are dwindling. They complain about the lack of engagement and commitment to the profession "these days", without taking a hard look at themselves and what they have actually accomplished over the many years of their existence. Most of these clubs are run by the same core group of individuals, slogging along trying to justify their existence by having monthly meetings, providing Continuing Education and another place for pharmacists to piss and moan.

Perhaps they would be better off reverting to the smoke filled, alcohol soaked meetings of old, where a pharmacist could join the rest of his gin blossomed cronies in a mutual commiseration session without feeling guilty for being a poor example.

FIGURE 4 INDIANA IPA WONDERS WHY IT CAN'T GET NEW MEMBERS

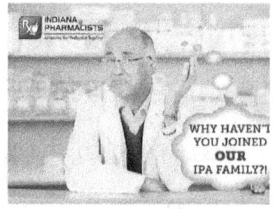

CHAPTER 14

BIG PHARMA

Big Pharma is the nickname given to the pharmaceutical industry and its trade group the Pharmaceutical Research and Manufacturers of America, or PhRMA. I'm not letting Big Pharma off the hook for their part in this whole fiasco. They have things to atone for, but an in- depth examination of the industry would probably fill another book. For now, suffice it to say that there have been numerous ethical lapses on the part of the pharmaceutical manufacturers, and their sales tactics and pricing structures are often suspect.

Although the industry has contributed to its own questionable reputation, there is much to be said for the advances in medical treatment that have become available to us in a relatively short time period. Consider that as recently as the Civil War (1861-1865), there were no antibiotics and no vaccines (other than the smallpox vaccine). Many deaths came as a result of infection or disease, rather than from the battle wounds themselves.

Pharmaceutical companies invest a significant amount of money in research and development, and there are no guarantees that the products they are working on will make it to the market. Don't get your Kleenex out for a pity party yet, though, because they have profited handsomely from their successes.

The global revenue for pharmaceutical companies was over $1 trillion in 2014, yet drug prices continue to rise, to the extent that some patients can no longer afford their medications. For

2017, drug prices for Americans under 65 were projected to rise 11.6 percent, while wages are only projected to rise 2.5 percent. Nobody argues with the fact that a company should make a fair profit when they take a risk and do the research to develop a new drug or improvement on an older drug. What is "fair" is what is in dispute.

This is one area that pharmacists could be of great benefit, if we were allowed to practice the way we want to practice. Sometimes it is possible to come up with a generic product, or a combination of generic products, that have the same therapeutic effect as a brand name or brand name combination products. I have a big problem with "me too" drugs, which are medications that are similar to a product that is already on the market. Sometimes, a new dosage form, such as a quick dissolve tablet or a liquid, can make it easier for patients to take their medication. At other times, "tweaking" an existing drug product is just a way to preserve market share.

FIGURE 5 TOP 10 U.S. PHARMACEUTICAL COMPANIES BY SALES:

COMPANY	2016	2015
Johnson & Johnson	$71.89 billion	$70.04 billion
Pfizer	$52.82 billion	$48.85 billion
Roche	$50.11 billion	$47.70 billion
Novartis	$48.52 billion	$49.41 billion
Merck & Co.	$39.8 billion	$39.5 billion
Sanofi	$36.57 billion	$36.73 billion

GlaxoSmithKline	$34.79 billion	$29.84 billion
Gilead	$30.39 billion	$32.15 billion
AbbVie	$25.56 billion	$22.82 billion
Bayer	$25.27 billion	$24.09 billion

The pharmaceutical companies wield a considerable amount of power politically. The industry employs 1378 paid lobbyists, and spent nearly $3.5 billion to influence politicians from the period 1998 to 2016, and spent about $246 million in 2016 alone. They also have a disturbing habit of doing what they want and paying the penalty later. (Drugwatch 2016)

CHAPTER 15

PHARMACISTS FIGHT BACK

Joseph W. Zorek, Rph of Harrisburg PA is my hero. While many pharmacists piss and moan and take abuse from their employers without retaliating, Joe put himself and his family in the line of fire, and took a stand against CVS pharmacy by filing a federal lawsuit in 2011 against the drugstore giant. Joe had worked for CVS for 44 years, with a sterling reputation and relationship with his patients, and an excellent record with regard to the running of his pharmacy department and pharmacy business metrics.

Joe has multiple sclerosis. MS inhibits Joe's ability to walk, and he has limited use of his right arm. Joe had worked for CVS for 21 years before being diagnosed with MS in 1989. Despite his condition, Joe had always run one of the top stores in the district, and he and his technicians worked well together. MS is a progressive disease, and as Joe began to experience more problems with mobility, he sought a way to accommodate his disability, since CVS never made any offer to help in this regard. He purchased a mobility chair, which worked well for him, until CVS, without consulting Joe, decided in 2007 to purchase an elevated office chair and required him to use it, stating that this would allow him to see over the counter and view the whole pharmacy area. The use of the chair actually made Joe's condition worse, and it made him feel like he had a neon sign advertising his disability.

When CVS began to cut technician hours, eventually slashing hours by 20%, Joe opposed the cuts, stating the obvious that reducing staff while increasing the pressure to put out more work would lead to errors and would endanger his patients. In May of 2011, the technician cuts were reversed, and Joe's store posted its highest ever corporate performance score.

By then, however, the winds of change were blowing. The suits began to pressure Joe to resign. This is a common tactic used by the chains when an experienced pharmacist, usually over 50 years of age, complains too loudly about issues regarding patient safety. If this angle does not work, they will use other means to force a resignation.

Joe's health suffered as a result of the constant harassment, and he went on disability leave in July of 2011. He filed a complaint with EEOC in October of that year, and in July of 2012, as the year of disability allowed by CVS expired, Joe was fired. (Penn Live.com 2013)

Joe sued CVS. CVS dragged out the proceedings by trying to get the case dismissed and used other stalling tactics, designed to wear Joe and his legal team down and prolong the process, hoping that Joe either ran out of money to fight, gave up and settled out of court, or was forced by deteriorating health to give up. It would not be a stretch to guess that they would not feel bad if Joe died before he got the satisfaction of seeing them punished for their abuses.

Joe fought on for 5 long years, refusing to settle, taking one for the team, hoping to win his case and finally bring to light the evil intentions and actions of the outwardly beneficent drug chains. As of this writing, there is no information online regarding the case after the date when Joe's attorneys submitted his request for a jury trial, filed January 31, 2014.

There are very few lawsuits filed by individual pharmacists that have succeeded. Two of the lucky ones, James King and Roger Harris, won their lawsuits against CVS and were awarded $1 million, and $400,000 respectively.

Mr. King was a CVS pharmacist working at a store located in Pell Alabama. He was hired in February 2004, and was fired on October 11, 2011. The harassment began in 2006, when Cody Berguson became King's pharmacy supervisor. Starting in late 2010, Berguson began to ask King "when are you going to retire" or "why don't you buy an annuity and retire". King reported the disparaging comments, and was subsequently suspended and then fired, allegedly for a prescription error, but in reality it was retaliation on the part of Berguson.

Mr. Harris was a 65 year old CVS pharmacist working in the same district in Alabama. He was fired shortly after he returned from a vacation celebrating his 65th birthday, and replaced by a 27 year old pharmacist. His district pharmacy supervisor had begun to call him "old man" and several other pharmacy employees began to follow suit. He was terminated on August 17, 2009. After a two -

week trial, a jury agreed with Harris and awarded him $400,000 in back, and $400,000 in damages. (Drug Topics 2015)

Dee Wigger was 58 years old when she filed a verified charge of discrimination with the Equal Employment Opportunity Commission (EEOC) on September 25, 2013. She received a Notice of Right to Sue from the EEOC on December 24, 2014. Ms. Wigger was hired by CVS in 1997. She worked as a staff pharmacist until 2010, when she was promoted to PIC (pharmacist in charge).

CVS began its Metrics program around 2008, and increased the requirements and pressure it put on its pharmacists to perform, mandating time to fill prescriptions, answer the phone, etc. Wigger continued to do well under these conditions, and had a positive relationship with her Pharmacy Supervisor and District Manager, always receiving high ratings on her performance evaluations.

When Darlene Mollet was hired as the new Pharmacy Supervisor in charge of Wigger's store in the fall of 2012, she became highly critical and hostile toward Wigger from the start. As a result of this mistreatment and the pressure of the ever - increasing pressure of the Metrics, Wigger was diagnosed by her psychiatrist with Post Traumatic Stress disorder and severe depression and took a leave of absence on his recommendation, starting in December 27, 2012 through the beginning of March 2013. When she returned to work, she was demoted to staff pharmacist and transferred to another location. Her position at her original location was filled by a younger, less experienced pharmacist. Her new PIC, "Millie" was hostile to Wigger and mistreated her, often screaming at her and telling her she had a reputation as a bad pharmacist.

Mollet began a systematic campaign to pressure Wigger and exacerbate her PTSD, fabricating outlandish stories and accusations, constantly riding her and writing her up for these fabricated accusations, and making her work environment unbearably hostile.

The account in the court documents illustrates the draconian tactics and extreme lengths chains like CVS and Walgreens will go to in their quest to eliminate older, more experienced pharmacists on the basis of Metrics (although younger pharmacists are unable to meet the Metrics, either). Once the older pharmacists are forced out, they can hire younger pharmacists for less pay and less experience to fill the vacated positions.

On August 27, 2013, under the direction of Darlene Mollet and District Manager Kevin Elliot, Wigger was fired and replaced with a younger, less experienced pharmacist. Her partner, PIC "Millie" was relegated to the floater pool at that same time, and she was also replaced by a younger, less experienced pharmacist. (CVS and 2:15-CV-01122-DCN-MGB 2014)

Another plaintiff was fired in retaliation for her complaints about safety conditions, and because of her gender. Maureen McPadden, a Walmart pharmacist won her wrongful termination case and was awarded $31 million. McPadden was fired in November of 2012, after working for Walmart for 13 years, allegedly for losing a pharmacy key. She suspected, however, that the real reason she was fired was because she claimed that customers at the Seabrook, New Hampshire store where she worked were getting improperly filled prescriptions because of inadequate staff training. The gender discrimination piece comes in because a male pharmacist had also lost a key, and he was not fired. McPadden's award included $15 million in punitive damages, $15 million in compensation for unlawful discrimination based on gender, and $750,000 in back pay. (Drug Topics 2016)

In any other arena, Jeremy Hoven would be hailed as a hero. In Walgreens World, such bravery will get you fired. At 4:30 in the morning on May 8th, the 36 year old Hoven was sorting medications behind the counter. Two armed men wearing masks entered the store, and immediately pointed their guns at one of the workers. They took a manager hostage, and dragged him through the aisles at gunpoint. Hoven tried to call 9-1-1. The second gunman had taken another manager hostage, and when he saw that Hoven was looking at him, he jumped over the pharmacy counter and fired at Hoven three times, but the gun missfired. Hoven pulled his own weapon in self-defense, firing 3 times at the robbers. They ran from the store in a panic.

Mr. Hoven was fired 5 days later, and filed a lawsuit against Walgreens, citing a Michigan law that allows citizens to defend themselves. Walgreens non-escalation policy, which forbids its pharmacists from carrying handguns, was used to defend their position. The judge sided with Walgreens in the case. (Good Morning America 2011)

Kelly Hoots, a CVS pharmacist in North Carolina, was fired for closing the drive thru during hour 7, in the midst of a 14 hour marathon shift, during which he had already filled 300 prescriptions (at a rate of 1 prescription every 84 seconds) with no food or bathroom breaks. Mr. Hoots made the decision to close the drive thru, as is his right as pharmacist in charge, because he was overwhelmed with the workload to the point where he couldn't properly counsel patients, a pharmacist duty that is strictly mandated by law. The store manager, a non- pharmacist, overrode his decision, and Mr. Hoots was fired over the incident. (Jim Plagakis 2011)

These cases illustrate why there is a culture of fear and a reluctance to speak out on the part of the pharmacists. It is rare for a pharmacist to win a lawsuit against one of these companies, even with careful documentation of the abuse and intimidation. Lawyers are reluctant to take these cases. At will employment protects the employers, and apparently even the most blatant and obvious mistreatment does not override this statute. The cases that are publicized have been picked up by the media and sensationalized, but in the underground blogs and forums, pharmacists share accounts of false accusations, slander, intimidation, hostile work environments, technician spies, write ups for not meeting Metrics, veiled threats and sarcastic comments about age and professional ability, nasty remarks about one's personal life, and general disrespect and mistreatment by employees and customers alike. Many pharmacists suffer from some form of depression or PTSD. Some become unable to work because of mental illness, and some commit suicide.

"I know 2 pharmacists that have already committed suicide. One in his 40s and one that was 26. I also know a few that went bonkers and quit and now don't do anything. I would say it's a combination of being undermined and working for a corporation that treats like you're not selling them enough t-shirts and you're an idiot that is easily replaceable to them.

There's also an ensuing personal battle that you're responsible for someone's health and medical needs and a job that expects you to do that as quickly as possible because being responsible or careful isn't measurable. I've had one friend that gave the wrong drug to someone that had an allergy and that person is in the hospital. The average pharmacists has less than 2 minutes to check their work or drugs...for 14 hours a day straight. That can be a start. Not to mention loans, self-worth, and whatever else is going on in that person's life." (Reddit 2014)

When pharmacists have acted as a group, they have been more successful in winning cases against the chains, but, unfortunately, the chains simply pay the judgements and move on. Nothing has changed, despite settlements in the millions of dollars. Apparently, this is the toll the chains are willing to pay to continue to steamroll over everyone who gets in the path of their business plan.

While pharmacists advocating for patient safety seem to disappear for nebulous reasons, the patients themselves are being treated like cogs in the medical machine. Occasionally, one must grease the palms of the masses when the system breaks down and one of them is hurt or killed, but one must do what one must do. If prescriptions are poison, let them eat cake.

CHAPTER 16

JUST ANOTHER COST OF DOING BUSINESS

Pharmacy is fraught with the potential for error by its very nature. We were taught in pharmacy school that there are no gray areas in pharmacy. It's black and white. Either it is right, or it isn't. Most pharmacists have some degree of OCD, which gives them an advantage when attention to detail and meticulous checking and rechecking are required. The kid who arranges his crayons in a specific color order in the box at 3 years old would probably make an excellent pharmacist.

The absolute worst thing that could ever happen to a pharmacist is to harm a patient. Even relatively minor prescription errors, including those that are caught in house and never even get to the patient, will cause the average pharmacist to lose sleep and beat themselves up for making a mistake.

Pharmacists hold patient lives in their hands every day. They dispense medications that are essentially poisons if prescribed or dosed improperly. Believe me when I tell you that the weight of that responsibility rests heavily on our shoulders. Keeping patients safe and not making errors is hard enough when the company has your back. When the company insists on making decisions that endanger patients, it becomes unbearable.

The individual pharmacist is expected to uphold the ethical and legal aspects of pharmacy practice, despite the fact that he often stands alone against the considerable force applied by his employer, unaided by anyone, including the state board of pharmacy or the government. Even his district pharmacy supervisor, who probably ascended to that position solely to get out from behind the bench, is silent when it comes to concerns about workload and patient safety.

While most pharmacies have a system for reporting errors in-house, this information is not required to be reported to outside agencies. Some pharmacists report every error, no matter how small, but some are reluctant to provide this information for fear of being disciplined or fired.

According the U.S. Food and Drug Administration, medication errors cause at least one death every day and injure 1.3 million people annually in the United States. This figure includes statistics from all areas of pharmacy practice, including hospital, long term care, and community pharmacy.

I'm not much on statistics. While it seems necessary to include them in a chapter about medication errors, 1.3 million people is an abstract concept to me. We are bombarded with statistics. Information overload leads to a lack of engagement with the real crux of the matters we are considering.

Statistics are cold and impersonal, and they do little to stir the emotions or compel anyone to take action. When I considered listing the numerous lawsuits and accounts of pharmacy errors and patient harm, I decided against it. The headlines and archives of newspapers and magazines are full of these accounts, and the internet fairly explodes with accounts of all manner of human misery that has been caused by medication errors.

What I am asking you to do instead is to focus on a friend, loved one, or acquaintance that has been harmed by a prescription or medical error, and to use their experience to inform your understanding of all that is wrong with the healthcare system. Let their hurt and anger affect you to the point that you are willing to put some effort into contacting the agencies that are responsible for the systems and conditions leading to these injuries and deaths.

I want to encourage and challenge you to put pressure on the people who have been given the power and responsibility to monitor the corporations and hold them accountable for putting patients in danger because of their greed and apathy. Fines, lawsuits, and settlements have become just another cost of doing business to the corporations who run our drug stores. Human life is apparently expendable, since absolutely no effort has been made to follow the advice and requests of pharmacists to make changes that would help keep patients safe.

I have included sample letters and contact information for the agencies and organizations responsible for overseeing the retail chain drug stores at the end of this book. I encourage you to use them.

Sometimes we feel powerless to make change happen. Considering the current situation in Washington, it is easy to get discouraged and feel like our voice doesn't matter. We have to find a way to overcome our cynicism and continue the fight anyway.

"There are a group of people who would like to silence everybody and have everybody go along to get along, but that's not going to be very helpful for us in the long run, in terms of solving our problems. And somebody has to be courageous enough to actually stand up to, you know, the bullies."
   Ben Carson

CHAPTER 17

BLOGS, ARTICLES, AND BOOKS

BY PHARMACISTS

Individual pharmacists have tried various tactics to get the word out about the danger to patients posed by the current pharmacy model. In this chapter, I will mention some of the more prominent pharmacist writers and bloggers who have been writing for years about staffing, metrics, and patient safety concerns. Despite the sustained efforts of these and other pharmacist writers to bring attention to the problems inherent in the retail pharmacy model, the fact remains that the only people who read their writings are other pharmacists. The general public, and even our relatives, are unable to grasp the magnitude of the problem, not only because they have never walked in our shoes, but also because, despite the barriers, most pharmacists do a very good job of keeping their patients safe, with the consequence that their own mental and physical health are compromised.

In 2013, I started a blog called "Behind the Counter, What Your Pharmacist Wishes You Knew" (http://bulldogpharmacist.blogspot.com).

I abandoned the blog after 23 posts, frustrated by the realization that I was preaching to the choir. Instead of patients, I was getting feedback from other pharmacists. While I enjoyed reading their comments, I had failed to reach the audience I was attempting to educate on ways to make their pharmacy experience easier and safer. I wanted to give the inside scoop and explain the reasons for some of the things we do in the pharmacy, and I wanted to explain that all of the things we do as individual pharmacists are motivated by a sense of responsibility and caring for our patients.

After what amounted to so much pissing in the wind, I doubled down on venting my frustrations through writing, and produced a series of 3 articles, which were published in Drug Topics Magazine in 2014. These articles are entitled "Who Will Stand up for Pharmacy", "A Dose of Pharmacy Truth, Report from the Front Lines" and "The Good, the Bad, and the Gray Areas, Where Are Your Ethics?". (http://drugtopics.modernmedicine.com/authorDetails/379211)

I also produced a You Tube video in 2014 entitled "Stand up for Pharmacy".

(https://www.youtube.com/watch?v=AhXHJgiNZP0&feature=youtu.beh)

Although the responses from other pharmacists were kind and encouraging, my goal of stirring them to action fell flat. And who was I kidding, sitting in my nice home office banging out my frustrations on the keys of my Mac, safe and secure in my new job, far away from Walgreens and the retail rat race.

There are many pharmacists out there who have given a more sustained effort to the cause than I, writing books, articles, blogs, and newsletters, as well as starting activist organizations, networking with other pharmacists, and trying to get the attention of the boards of pharmacy and government officials. Some brave souls have even sued their former employers for wrongful termination, a particularly life sucking prospect, given its David and Goliath-esc proportions.

Pharmacist Jim Plagakis, a staunch advocate of better and safer working conditions, and a no nonsense, straight talking hero of the profession, started writing his column "JP at Large" for Drug Topics Magazine in 1989. For years, his was the only voice that spoke the truth, taking the powers that be and the pharmacists themselves to task for what he rightly perceived as a profession being taken over by the chains.

Drug Topics Magazine is to be commended for its tradition of providing a platform for pharmacists to speak out about topics that are forbidden anywhere else. (Drug Topics- Voice of the Pharmacist)

While privately, pharmacists looked forward to JP's columns and applauded his ability to write what they all were thinking, publicly, they smiled and nodded and complied every time the corporate goons came up with some new way to screw them, preferring to continue to wear the Golden Handcuffs and reap short term gains rather than accept responsibility and risk losing their nice income and the delusion that they were still respected professionals.

JP also started what I refer to affectionately as a renegade pharmacy group called The Pharmacist Alliance (TPA) which later morphed into the more militaristic sounding Guerilla Pharmacist.

Jim's messages were simple and direct: "A Tired Pharmacist is a Dangerous Pharmacist", "Document, document, document, and, if forced to do so, "Sue the Bastards". His books (The Prisoners of Comfort, The Rebels of Comfort, and The Dangerous Book for Pharmacists) are nothing less than a call to arms, meant to spur a literal revolution in our profession.

Jim's health has frequently put him out of commission for long periods of time, but he has always come fighting back, ready to take on the powers that be and expose their abuses of pharmacists and the public. He deserves to rest on his laurels, secure in the knowledge that he has been a source of comfort and inspiration to thousands of us over the many years he has bravely advocated for the profession.

Pharmacist Steve Ariens is another long- time advocate of the profession, and co-founder of TPA. He continues to blog, network, and push for change. He is particularly involved in advocating for pain management patients who have been stigmatized by the opiate addiction crises and who have difficulty getting their prescriptions filled. We will discuss pain management and the opioid epidemic in a later chapter. Steve's website, pharmaciststeve.com, lists most of the other pharmacy blogs under the section entitled "What Pharmacist Steve is Reading". A list of these blogger sites is included in the Appendix.

I feel the need to caution those who are interested in reading some of the pharmacy blogs. The blogs are not written with the public in mind. They are sometimes raw, angry, and often profane. Anyone who is not a pharmacist may be shocked to see how customers are portrayed and discussed in these un-sanitized forums. It is probably too much to ask, but perhaps seeing things from the other side of the counter might give patients some insight into what the pharmacy staff has to deal with behind the scenes.

Pharmacist and former CVS employee Dee Wigger runs a Facebook page called "Pharmacists United for Change" which currently has only 133 members. It is a closed group, whose purpose is to post updates about legislation, lawsuits, and abuses committed by the chains and other pharmacy corporations.

Pharmacist Dennis Miller has long been a voice of the profession. He has written scores of articles for Drug Topics Magazine and other publications. His books, "Pharmacy Exposed: 1,000 Things That Can Go Deadly Wrong at the Pharmacy", and "Chain Drug Stores are Dangerous" How Their Reckless Obsession with the Bottom Line Places You at Risk for Serious Harm or Death" are clear about the evils of retail chains.

One would think that the titles alone would scare the bejesus out of the public, but unfortunately, of the 28 reviews I found listed for his "Pharmacy Exposed" book, and the 4 reviews listed for "Chain Drug Stores are Dangerous", most, if not all, of the reviews are from fellow pharmacists. The population he most wanted to reach has for some reason ignored his books, despite their alarming titles. Perhaps the huddled masses are simply too overwhelmed by the mass buggery they are subjected to on a daily basis to read one more account of why they should be upset about their unfortunate situation with regard to safety at the pharmacy.

Daniel A. Hussar Ph.D. publishes a newsletter called The Pharmacist Activist, which leads off each month with a pointed discussion of issues, and ends with a nice update on new medications and therapies. He continues to speak out regularly on behalf of pharmacists, most of whom are too cowed by their employers to say anything that might spark retaliation. Dr. Hussar has served the profession well, and has acted in many capacities to the benefit of the profession. (Pharmacy Times 2017)

I recently discovered a relative newcomer to the scene when I began listening to podcasts on a daily basis. Alex Barker, along with former park ranger Jody Mayberry, teamed up to produce a podcast in 2016 on Pharmacy Life Radio that promised to "Make Your Life 10% Better". I don't know about my life, but it definitely makes my day at least 10% better when I hear this energetic 30 something's ideas for taking your pharmacy career into your own hands and carving out your own niche in the profession, practicing pharmacy the way it was meant to be practiced.

He says the book "The 7 Habits of Highly Effective People" by Stephen Covey changed his life. He is on track to change some lives himself, if he continues to produce content like this.

There are many talented pharmacists who write for publications like Drug Topics and Pharmacy Times. The articles in these magazines are generally for pharmacists only, but a quick perusal of some of the content might prove enlightening for the lay person.

CHAPTER 18

THE OPIOID EPIDEMIC

"Trump declares opioid crisis a national emergency!" the headlines scream. Well, duh.

Opium and morphine addiction have been around for centuries. Man has sought to relieve his physical and psychic pain through the use and abuse of intoxicating substances since the beginning of his existence. Life is difficult, and who can blame people for trying to ease some of the misery, if relief can be found in the ingestion of a plant or chemical substance? Show me someone who claims they would never become addicted to pain medication, and I'll show you someone who is either lying, or who has not experienced the level of pain that brings a patient to the brink or commission of suicide.

Pain management is tricky, not only because every patient responds differently to pain medications, but also because pain has a huge psychological component. There is no way to predict how a patient is going to react or respond. Thus, these patients require intense monitoring and support, but they should not be denied a medication that relieves their pain.

Some doctors claim that the sales tactics of the pharmaceutical companies that started to escalate in the 1990's induced them to start writing more prescriptions for these powerful drugs. They say that the pharmaceutical sales reps falsely claimed that the new narcotics coming out on the market were not addictive, and that this is the reason they started writing more prescriptions for drugs like Perdue Pharma's Oxycontin. This argument does not hold water, however, since every doctor has been taught and should be aware that these substances are addictive, given the right circumstances, in any individual patient.

If a sales rep has the ability to influence doctors to ignore the lessons of history and their clinical training, then sign me up for some of that power. I would love to have somebody listen to my professional opinion on the matter. Hell, I'd love to have somebody listen to anything I have to say about anything.

A word about addiction, since "the Opiate Crises" is now upon us. Pharmacists have been seeing the results of addiction and drug seeking behavior for years, but since the politicians didn't have to see what was happening to patients, they didn't want to be bothered. Now, all of a sudden, it's the talk of the town. Everybody and their brother seems to have an answer to the problem, but most of the people running their mouths have no idea what they are talking about, nor do they care, as long as it sounds good and gets them reelected.

The real drug experts are too busy coping with the shit storm that has occurred as a result of our broken healthcare system, too mired down in regulations, employer mandates, and distractions to band together and work on the problems in a constructive way. So far, the government has focused on punishment rather than treatment. Obviously, this approach has failed miserably.

Beginning in 1971, Nixon's "war on drugs" provided a handy reason to scapegoat and target groups who were inconvenient to the government at the time. In 1994, reporter Dan Baum tracked down John Erlichman, a top Nixon aide, and questioned him about the antidrug campaign:

"You want to know what this was really all about. The Nixon campaign in 1968, and the Nixon White House after that, had two enemies: the antiwar left and black people. You understand what I'm saying? We knew we couldn't make it illegal to be either against the war or black, but by getting the public to associate the hippies with marijuana and the blacks with heroin, and then criminalizing both heavily, we could disrupt those communities. We could arrest their leaders, raid their homes, break up their meetings, and vilify them night after night on the evening news. Did we know we were lying about the drugs? Of course we did." (Harper's 2016)

The war on drugs apparently did not extend to medications prescribed by a doctor, and the perception of the public was that these drugs were safe to use, since they were not "street drugs". My mother, an ICU nurse and a no nonsense straight shooter, once spoke up in a Sunday School class full of fine Methodist Christians and got herself kicked out of the class. The subject was "kids these days" and "drug abuse" and "smoking marijuana". After listening to the outrage and horror expressed vociferously by several class members, Mom simply asked how many of these upstanding members of the community had a bottle of Valium or other "mother's little helpers" in their possession, and how many of them took medication to calm their nerves. Crickets. I guess nobody wanted to talk about those particular drugs.

Soon after Ronald Reagan took office in 1981, Nancy Reagan began her "Just Say No" campaign. This campaign was the forerunner of the zero tolerance policies instituted in the 1980's, which lead to a massive increase in incarcerations. During this era, the DARE drug education program was started in the nation's schools, although the program showed little evidence that it was effective in stopping kids from using drugs.

In the late 1980's and early 1990's, laws were passed that further increased the prison population. The American public became convinced that drug abuse was the nation's number one problem, and that harsher drug policies were the answer. President Clinton spoke of treatment over imprisonment during his campaign, but then did nothing during his time in office to promote this idea.

During George W Bush's tenure, more money was allocated to the war on drugs, and enforcement became more militarized, resulting in SWAT team raids on American citizens at the rate of 40,000 per year. Many of these raids were for non - violent drug offenses and misdemeanors.

These federal mandates began to be softened by the states, until public opinion has now shifted to favoring a health based approach to drug abuse rather than criminalization. With overdose deaths on the rise, many states passed "911 Good Samaritan" laws and increased access to naloxone, an injectable drug that counteracts narcotics overdoses.

President Obama , although in favor of shifting the majority of drug policy from criminalization to a health based approach, was unable to influence lawmakers to join him in this endeavor.

The current administration wants to go back to the drug wars of the 1980s. Attorney General Jeff Sessions does not support state sponsored legalization of marijuana, and has made this statement:

"Good people don't smoke marijuana."
Which can only mean one thing. Trump and his cabinet members must be major tokers. (Drug Policy Alliance 2017)

Addiction, whether psychological or physical, or both, is often thought to be a moral failing on the part of an individual who is too weak to resist medicating himself to cope with life. In reality, this need to find relief from the stresses and strains of life is a universal need that all humans have. If you have found solace in legal substance abuse, by drinking alcohol, smoking, or taking prescription drugs, or if you have developed another form of addiction to distract yourself from the pit hole of hell that life represents, recognize that there but for the grace of God go you.

New studies indicate that, not only is addiction not a moral failing on the part of the individual, but in reality all humans have the potential to become addicted to opiates and other substances, or even behaviors, given the right circumstances. While there is some evidence for a genetic link to addiction, the crux of the problem is not the drug itself, nor is the need or desire to seek relief from pain. Addiction occurs when the brain starts to associate the ingestion of the drug with pleasure. When the pleasure center is activated, any behavior can become addictive, including exercise, eating, sex, video gaming, or even organizing and cleaning.

In his excellent book "Irresistible", Adam Alter points out that our obsession with electronic devices has produced a population that is literally addicted to screen time to the detriment of themselves and society. He states that while Apple touted the wonders of the IPad, Steve Jobs would not even let his children have an IPad. The full effect of this technology on the brains of our children is yet to be seen.

Alter goes on to discuss the origins of other addictions, citing the case of a lab rat with a metal electrode implanted in the pleasure center of his brain. The rat learned that every time he pressed a metal bar in his cage, an electric shock stimulated this pleasure center. The rat soon became so addicted to pressing the bar that he stopped eating and drinking and eventually died from exhaustion. (Alter 2017)

In my recollection, one of the main reasons opioids began to become prescribed more freely in the 1990's had more to do with the basics of pain relief, rather than the aforementioned army of opioid pushing sales reps.

In 1986, the WHO published its "three step analgesic ladder", which was meant to be used to address the pain experienced by HIV and cancer patients. There had been several studies done that showed that many cancer patients were not getting adequate doses of narcotics to control their pain because of concerns about them becoming addicted. The studies also found that patients who were allowed to experience severe pain in between doses had a harder time getting pain relief than patients whose pain was kept at a reasonable level. This "remembered pain" is described as the brain's memory of past pain in certain circumstances, and the anticipation of a repeat occurrence of that pain, given the same circumstances. If you have ever had extensive dental work done, you will understand this phenomenon.

This knowledge led to the use of a long acting narcotic, like Oxycontin, backed up by a faster acting, shorter duration narcotic like oxycodone for breakthrough pain, or pain not controlled by the Oxycontin. Doctors were urged not to worry about the risk of addiction in cancer patients, but to focus instead on keeping them as comfortable as possible.

The upshot was that once the floodgates were opened, the use of this narcotic regimen began to be applied to all kinds of pain, including back pain, tooth pain, migraines, post-surgical pain, and many other types of acute and chronic pain which had been more conservatively treated in the past by drugs like acetaminophen, ibuprofen and other NSAIDS, and milder, smaller doses of narcotics if necessary.

As narcotic prescriptions became easier to issue, unscrupulous physicians started to creep out of the underbrush to capitalize on the otherwise legitimate use of these medications.

The drugs became available on the street, and their escalating street value led some people to turn to heroin, which is cheaper, and one of the most dangerous drugs on the planet.

Whether the writing of ever higher doses and quantities of opioids stems from a place of empathy for the patient in pain, lack of resources for the supervision and support of the patient, or simply unmitigated greed, the result is the same. You now have a person who is addicted to a substance that keeps them coming back to you for ever higher doses and quantities, because, over time, they develop tolerance, and the dose must be raised to provide the same effect.

The patients who develop physical and psychological addictions to these medications have few options for assistance when it comes to weaning down to the lowest effective dose or augmenting medication with therapies like acupuncture, massage, physical therapy, and psychological counseling. A multidisciplinary approach is what is needed, but these interventions take time, and modern society does not allow for such luxuries. Instead, people are patched up with pills and sent home, or back to work. A lucky few have good insurance, money to pay the copays, short or long- term disability coverage, and understanding employers. Their home life is safe and supportive, and they have people in their lives who care about them and assist them in addressing their health issues. When these things are not in place, the patient's stress is magnified, adding to his perception of pain, both physical and psychological, and leading to desperate attempts to get relief at any cost.

The goal should be keeping the patient comfortable with the lowest dose of pain medication possible by assisting them in understanding the causes of pain, supporting them and giving them the tools they need to manage their pain, and taking the time to listen and make adjustments to their treatment plan as necessary. This approach takes time, money, energy, and reorganization of the healthcare system into a cooperative, multidisciplinary team, instead of the current disjointed, competitive and largely ineffective system we have now. God forbid healthcare professionals are enabled to practice at the top of their licenses and apply their full range of knowledge and energy to the problem. What a radical concept.

Pharmacists have seen their inventory of narcotics increase exponentially over the years, necessitating more and larger narcotic cabinets, along with tighter "security" (more on that later), and more restrictions on the dispensing of narcotics and controlled substances.

They were there to see the beginning of the opioid epidemic and continue to see the struggle many patients have with addiction. They have seen the story play out time after time.

The story goes something like this:

Sam is a hard worker. He works in a steel mill 7 days a week. Sam is approaching 50, and his body is beginning to show signs that the heavy lifting and extreme heat are starting to take their toll. His old shoulder injury from his time in Iraq has started to flare up and become more of a hindrance. So far, Sam has self-medicated with a beer or six after work, and he goes through a case of Budweiser every weekend.

One day, Sam bends over to pick something up off the floor, and his back goes out. His buddy takes him to the ER, the doctor examines him, tells him he has a slipped disc, and writes a prescription for Oxycontin 10mg twice a day, #30, and Vicodin, 1-2 tablets every 4-6 hours as needed for breakthrough pain. He tells Sam to follow up with his family doctor or a chiropractor. He suggests an ice pack, alternating with a heating pad for 24 hours if possible.

After some time off and a month of light duty, Sam's pain has diminished somewhat, but it is always present. He doesn't want to go on disability just because of a slipped disc. He goes to his family doctor, who refers him to a pain specialist after the many prescriptions he has written for pain have failed to provide relief for Sam. At the pain clinic, the waiting room is full of blue collar working people like him, and a few people who have obviously been severely injured in an accident or who have had surgery. He fills out the forms and waits until he is eventually called in to see the doctor. After he examines Sam, the doctor writes for Oxycontin 10mg twice a day, with Vicodin for breakthrough pain. Sam explains that this dose is not cutting it for his now chronic back pain, so the doc increases the dose to 20mg twice a day and tells Sam to return in two weeks. He also writes for a physical therapy consult, but Sam knows he can't make the appointments or the copays, so he tosses the order in the trash on his way out of the office.

Sam does return to the pain clinic doctor, with the news that his bosses have mandated overtime to meet the demand of an increase in orders. Sam tells the doctor that his wife is pissed at him for working all the time, but that she also doesn't see the need to stick to a budget. He rarely sees his kids, and he is missing out on their sporting events. He knows they will soon be going to college, and the realization depresses him and weighs on his mind. On top of that, the damn pills aren't working, and he can't sleep without drinking a few beers before bedtime. The doctor tells him it is dangerous to mix narcotics with alcohol, and Sam says he just wants something that takes care of the pain. The doctor writes for Oxycontin 40mg twice a day, and replaces the Vicodin with oxycodone 5mg every 4 to 6 hours as needed for pain, with a stern warning to stop drinking alcohol with the pills. This dose seems to do the trick, and Sam feels much better.

As if someone turned off a spigot, the overtime suddenly dries up. There are rumors of layoffs, and Sam's hours are cut to 40 hours per week, with no overtime allowed. Three months later, the mill announces it is closing up and moving to Mexico by the end of the year. Six months after that, Sam receives his final paycheck from the steel mill. Now Sam is home all the time. He wonders why he missed his kids, because they have become surly and belligerent, and they are a pain in the ass. They don't speak to him voluntarily, except to ask for money. His wife is bitchy and nags him all the time. He has invaded her space all of a sudden, and she is not coping well. He finds excuses to go out to the garage or outside to putter around to avoid her discontent. They are not having sex, and he is so pissed at his wife, he doesn't really care. Every time money is mentioned, there is a huge fight. They have never been on the same page financially, but it didn't seem worth the conflict when Sam was working all the overtime and was able to bring home good money. Now he is collecting unemployment, along with his military pension, and the only jobs available for someone his age and with his abilities is Home Depot or Lowe's, and he'll be goddamned if he'll wear a stupid vest and kiss customer's asses for 10 dollars an hour.

Sam starts to take a few extra Oxy's now and then, washed down with a beer. He notices that he is more relaxed and less likely to explode when his wife or kids piss him off. As a matter of fact, when he gets a good buzz going, he could care less about his family or anything else. It's not his fault he got hurt at work, and his family never appreciated how hard he worked anyway, just wanted more and more. He deserves an escape. God knows he can't afford a nice family vacation, which would probably be a disaster anyway, and his wife would make his life miserable if he went on a fishing trip with his buddies. So, he takes a vacation in his mind.

Soon, Sam is spending most of his time on the couch watching T.V. or surfing the net. His wife and kids go about their business, and don't seem to mind that he is not involved in their lives. He has lost his identity as a man, and he feels like he has let his family down. He has nothing to be proud of anymore. The only people who understand him are his buddies from work, and the guys down at the VFW, and they all have their own problems. When they do get together, all they do is drink and bitch. Sam drives home from these liquid therapy sessions along the back roads. The last thing he needs right now is to get picked up for a DUI.

  The pharmacist at the local Walgreens is starting to give Sam a hard time every time he brings in his prescriptions to be filled. He threatens to take his business elsewhere, but it seems like too much of a hassle. The pharmacist even calls his doctor and questions him about Sam's medicine. Sam thinks this is between him and his doctor, and is none of this son of a bitch's business. The pharmacist's job is to fill the prescriptions, plain and simple. How long could it take to count a few pills and put them in a bottle? Sam doesn't want to make two trips, so he sits and waits in the cheesy waiting room and watches the other customers. The pharmacist seems to be the only person back there. After 45 minutes, he starts to get pissed and asks what the holdup is. The pharmacist explains that he is waiting for the doctor at the pain clinic to call him back, because he has a question about Sam's medication. When Sam asks why, the pharmacist says he is concerned that Sam is wanting his medication early, and he needs *to make sure his doctor is aware that he just got a 30 day supply 27 days ago.*

"Are you fucking kidding me? Give me my goddamn prescriptions back, I'll take them to CVS!" Sam storms out of the store, jumps in his truck, and lays rubber in the parking lot.

And so it goes. Sam's new job becomes spending time on the phone, in the doctor's office, and at the pharmacy, trying to get his prescriptions filled. Somebody from his work mentions that he knows a guy that can get Sam Oxy if he wants it. So far, Sam has avoided purchasing narcotics off the street, but if this keeps up, he may have to go that route.

Stories like this are common. Ordinary people, living ordinary lives, until something happens to them and they need to be treated for pain. Then they become labeled, the supply of narcotics suddenly begins to be restricted or dries up completely, and the person becomes desperate. Some turn to buying narcotics on the street. Others find doctors who are willing to write prescriptions and exploit these patients for financial gain. When the supply or the money dries up, many turn to the cheaper and more dangerous heroin for relief.

The CDC released Guidelines for Prescribing Opiates for Chronic Pain in 2016. The guide is intended for healthcare professionals, and it is long and complicated, but its intent is "to improve communication between clinicians and patients about the risks and benefits of opioid therapy for chronic pain, improve the safety and effectiveness of pain treatment, and reduce the risks associated with long-term opioid therapy, including opioid use disorder, overdose, and death." (Dowell D 2016)

The individual states have instituted prescription monitoring programs (PMP) to track the use of opioid prescriptions, and to share this information with other states in order to prevent "doctor shopping" and early refills on prescriptions for controlled substances. In Indiana, the program is called INspect. Pharmacies and pharmacists register for access to the program, and after they set up an online profile, they can look up a patient's history of controlled substance prescriptions. The database is searchable by name, address, aliases, connections with other persons or family members, etc. The search will bring up the drug, strength, quantity, date of fill, and the name of the pharmacy where the prescription was filled (name, location, and phone number). The database is helpful in tracking the use of controlled substances, and is reported to have decreased opioid overdose deaths in states with robust prescription drug monitoring programs as compared to states with weaker PMPs. (Pardo 2017)

Walgreens controversial Good Faith Dispensing Policy, or GFD, (see Appendix) requires a search of the PMP database, as well as a search of the history of prescriptions for controlled substances for all of the Walgreens stores in the chain. Patients and physicians complain that the policy is too intrusive and interferes with the physician/patient relationship. Patients consider it "none of our business" and doctors don't like pharmacists questioning their prescribing habits.

However, the new mandates were put in place only after years and years of abuses like doctor shopping, pill mills, and drug diversion, dirty doctors and pharmacists, and dishonest patients trying to gain the system. These procedures obviously increase the time it takes to process prescriptions for controlled substances. Unfortunately, as with all laws forced on the general population, they affect every patient, physician, and pharmacist, not just the ones who are doing bad things.

I practiced in retail pharmacy in one capacity or another (clinic, small independent chain, large retail chain) from 1989 to 2013. Most of the time I worked in Ft Wayne and the surrounding areas, although I did cover some shifts in in Peru, Marion, Logansport, Wabash, Huntington, and Portland during my years with Walgreens. From 1989 to 1999, I remember certain patients who tried to get their controlled substances filled early, or who altered or tried to call in their own prescriptions, but they were few and far between. At one time, we were allowed to dispense schedule V controlled substances like THC (terpin hydrate with codeine cough syrup), Robitussin with codeine, and Paregoric (for diarrhea) with a patient's signature, and we had a few problems with drug seekers trying to obtain these substances from multiple pharmacies, but it was not a significant part of our day There were a few well known "Dr. Goods" in the area, but not many, and I don't recall dealing with "pain clinics" at that time.

From 2000 on, there was not only a gradual increase in prescribed narcotics, but also an increase in pharmacy robberies. The relationship of the pharmacist with the patients began to deteriorate, and became more and more antagonistic. Much of this was due to the changes imposed by insurance companies, when they began to restrict formularies and require prior authorizations for non-generic and expensive medications, but there was also a shift in the type and number of patients being prescribed narcotics for pain.

In the past, the only patients who got regular prescriptions for potent narcotics were cancer patients and patients with severe disability from accidents or chronic disease. We began to see patients with back pain and neck pain, fibromyalgia, and migraines, as well as various other nonspecific and generalized pain syndromes which were unsuccessfully treated by other means like NSAIDS, steroids, and injections.

One of the early pioneers of pain management theory was Dr. John Bonica, an Army surgeon during WWII, who wrote "The Management of Pain" published in 1953. His book introduced the concept of a multidisciplinary, multi modal approach to pain, and was based on his experiences treating war veterans for chronic pain. As time went on, it became clear that pain was a complex, multifaceted phenomenon, which involved not only somatic or physical pain, and the perception of this pain in the cerebral cortex, but also what might be termed psychological pain, which is affected by emotions, living conditions, beliefs, attitudes, social support, and psychological perceptions. The new approach to pain management was termed the "biopsychosocial" approach, for want of a better word. (Johnson n.d.)

The Mayo Clinic pioneered one of the first pain management practices beginning in 1974. Dr. Lee Nauss joined Mayo at that time, and although his training was in regional anesthesia, he introduced epidural steroid injections, which became so popular with patients that he soon opened a stand-alone pain clinic and recruited Dr Tony Wang to run the clinic. Intrathecal morphine injections were one of the early therapies studied in this clinic. The tradition of anesthesiologists practicing pain management on the side began to be replaced by dedicated pain management practices. (PubMed 2011)

While there is certainly enough blame to go around, and patients themselves are the ones ultimately responsible for educating themselves and taking control of their own healthcare, it is the responsibility of the healthcare team to help the patient understand their condition and guide them toward a best-case scenario with regard to their medication therapy. It makes me angry that physicians have been given free rein to prescribe and overprescribe narcotics for years, while pharmacists have been expected to be the gate keepers of all controlled substances, with the ultimate responsibility for patient harm or death. Pharmacists are held responsible if a patient is injured or killed, but we are also held responsible if we "deny treatment" that is prescribed by the physician and requested by the patient.

The physicians stonewall us when we call to get the patients' condition and reason for the use of the medication, the patients get angry and tell us we have no business questioning them or their doctor, and our employers require us to give every patient the third degree on every single prescription for a controlled substance, while putting pressure on us to make every single patient happy.

Once again, we are in the unenviable position of being liable for decisions made by others who we do not control. We are denied the necessary information to evaluate these decisions, and we are not empowered with the legal authority to override these decisions. We stand between the physician and the patient with no legal authority, no respect, and no protection should the patient become upset or violent. Yet, we are to use our "professional judgement".

One of the major causes of pharmacist burnout is this mandate that we make everybody happy but do no harm. We have no authority, but all of the responsibility, and the whore mongers and physicians like it this way.

Things the pharmacist must not do:

"Don't offend the physician, for he writes the prescriptions we fill"
"Don't offend the patient, for he chooses which pharmacy to use"
"Don't offend the receptionist or the office nurses, for they are the gateway to the doctor"

"Don't ask too many questions and interfere in the doctor/patient relationship"

"Don't ask too few questions and miss an interaction or dosing error."

"Don't fill a prescription that causes patient harm"

"Don't deny a prescription to a patient who needs it"

"Don't make the patient wait too long"

"Don't neglect the other patients waiting for prescriptions or make them wait"

"Don't make an error, and don't miss the errors made by others"

Things the pharmacist must do:

"Do have prescriptions ready within 30 minutes or less"

"Do remain pleasant and calm

"Do maintain razor sharp focus and accuracy"

"Do make insurance claims go through, but don't commit fraud"

"Do perform proper research and exert maximum vigilance over opioid use and abuse"

"Do prevent overuse of opioids and controlled substances"

"Do keep the patient safe and counsel them properly"

Apparently, we are not worthy of respect, authority, or a position on the healthcare team, until it becomes convenient or necessary to find a patsy to send out as a whipping boy. Then, suddenly we become the "drug experts" and "knew or should have known" and "should have used our professional judgement". I contend that I can't use my professional judgement unless I am treated like a professional all of the time, not just when it becomes convenient to assign blame for something that is out of my control.

CHAPTER 19

THE GREAT FLU SHOT SCAM

The answer most companies put forth when asked why their CEO's and executives make such high salaries, is that it takes that kind of money to attract top notch individuals who are qualified to lead a large corporation successfully. If pay for performance is key, however, these guys just aren't cutting it.

According to insiders.morningstar.com, in 2016, Key Executives of Walgreens Boots Alliance received $38, 397,373 in total compensation, while their stock price dropped 50.54%. CVS Key Executives raked in $42, 652, 403, as their stock price dropped 23.33 %. Not to be outdone, Rite Aid, the side piece recently denied to poor Walgreens, paid Key Executives $44,878,394 to reward their investors with a whopping 58.81% drop in stock price.

It has not been a good decade for the drug store biz. Insurance companies and PBM's have cut reimbursements to pharmacies. Drug companies have raised prices. This has caused corporate management to look for other ways to make money in the pharmacies. The Big Boys (for they are almost exclusively men), put on their thinking caps and pondered, "what to do, what to do?".

In standard fashion, they went after the largest expense categories, which are inventory and payroll. They cut inventory to the bone, cut hours, cut staff, fired or pushed out older, higher paid (and experienced) pharmacists and brought in recent grads with huge ($250,000) student loans. They paid them less, and kept them below the required number of hours to be eligible for benefits. Not only were these young pharmacists in debt, they were also easier to manage, since they did not have the benefit of years of experience when dealing with their corporate overlords. They were eager to please in their new jobs, and, for the most part, they went along with whatever was asked of them without complaint. With the old gray mares out to pasture, the thoroughbreds were in the traces and ripe for the whipping. Too bad the old Conestoga's they pulled were outdated and in need of repair.

 Looking back the wheels began to fall off the wagons in earnest in 2008, when the now ubiquitous immunizations first reared their ugly head. Flu shots were the forerunner for all of the subsequent vaccines we would eventually be required to give to patients. Advertisements for the newly available service expressed the chain pharmacy's concern for the patients and their families. The flu could kill people. Everybody should get a flu shot as soon as possible. How convenient, to simply stop by your local drug store any time the pharmacy was open and quickly get that flu shot out of the way.

 Coincidentally, 2008 was also the year of the Avian flu scare, the much -heralded pandemic that was supposed to wipe out 150 million people if it struck. It didn't, but the scary headlines provided free advertising for the chains, who couldn't believe their luck. (nytimes.com, Jan. 22, 2008).

A little side story on the subject of the Avian flu scare. In 2008, I was sent by my pharmacy manager to attend an emergency meeting being held by Dr. Deborah McMahon, Health Commissioner for the Fort Wayne, Allen County Department of Health. The meeting was a call to arms for healthcare professionals to volunteer to help the community, should the Avian flu epidemic become a reality. The meeting was attended by about 20 to 30 pharmacists, nurses, and other healthcare workers. We were informed that the decision had been made to use the War Memorial Coliseum to house and isolate victims of the virus in order to help stem the spread of the illness, as well as to provide basic care for the needs of the patients.

Dr. McMahon had compiled a list of medications she wanted in an emergency kit, and she asked the pharmacists to help coordinate the assembly, labeling, and distribution of the kits, no small task, as you may imagine. She then went on to say that, since there is really nothing to be done for flu victims except to provide comfort and try to keep them hydrated throughout the course of the illness, volunteers would be needed to tend to the patients occupying the massive Coliseum, the local venue for big name concerts, Sports Vacation and Boat Shows, and the like.

My problem with the meeting was not with the plan itself, but with the fact that pharmacists, who are generally disrespected and treated as the red headed step children of the healthcare establishment, were all of a sudden valuable members of the healthcare team when the time came to put together God knows how many emergency kits (which may or may not be used) figure out how to get them donated or paid for, and be on hand to not only help administer the medications (a task that could be performed by anyone), but also to help perform basic tasks like cleaning up shit and vomit, bathing patients, and changing the bedding of the potentially thousands of victims lined up in the temporary isolation ward. Apparently, Dr. McMahon had heard about our reputation as the Whores of Healthcare.

Anyway, back to the flu shot scam. At first, immunization training for pharmacists was voluntary. It soon became mandatory, however, as the chains saw their sales begin to rise in tandem with the number of flu shots administered. Whether this revenue was from the shots themselves, or just an increase in foot traffic, is up for debate. Either way, the flu shots were key. At Walgreens, immunization training was conducted in 2 days, about 4 hours per session. The first day consisted of an Immunization Certified pharmacist reading the training material out loud to a room full of pharmacists as they followed along with their own copies.

At the end of Day 1, the pharmacists were shown the technique for an IM and ID (intradermal) injection, gave one of each type of shot to a partner, and class was dismissed. On Day 2, a written exam was administered, with the trainer reading each question aloud and giving "helpful hints" to ensure that all the pharmacists passed the exam and became certified. After giving an IM (intramuscular) and an ID (intradermal) injection in front of the trainer, the pharmacist received a link to print out a certificate on their computer, and the training was complete. Each pharmacist was now "Immunization Certified" and was authorized to give any and all vaccines allowed by the state they were licensed in.

There was also a separate CPR class given by a Red Cross certified trainer, which ran the pharmacists through basic CPR and included a practical and written exam on the same day. The pharmacists were required to keep this certification current and attend refresher classes every two years.

The set up for giving immunizations varied, but in my store, the station consisted of a card table covered with a cheap white plastic tablecloth from the party aisle, 2 rickety plastic chairs from the break room, an emergency kit comprised of a tote containing 2 adult Epi Pens and a Pediatric Epi pen, a CPR mask taped to the wall, and a blood pressure cuff.

For privacy, there was a screen with three panels of the type often used as a room divider, which allowed a full view of the patient from certain angles. This screen was of course adorned with Walgreens ads depicting happy, well rested pharmacists leisurely giving immunizations to smiling customers. Some stores had a private immunization room set up, but since the pharmacist often worked alone, this left the pharmacy unoccupied, which is both against the law and leaves the other patients in the lurch.

In the beginning, we gave flu shots when the customers came in to the store and asked for a flu shot. As time went on, the Store Manager began to bug us about asking people if they wanted a flu shot. This escalated to the point that I actually had to sign a paper that said I promised to ask "each and every patient if they would like a flu shot today." I lied and signed the damn paper, but I had no intention of harassing my patients for Walgreens benefit.

Despite their altruistic utterances, the real reason chain pharmacies care so very much if you get a flu shot every year boils down to the same reason they do anything: money. Pharmacies generally administer flu shots for around $32. Each dose costs the company between $9.50 and $16.72. In 2011, Walgreens brought 5.5 million people through their doors for flu shots. Not only did this increase their pharmacy sales, but it also helped boost their out- front profits by increasing foot traffic. (Info Wars 2012)

The next vaccine to be promoted was Zostavax, the shingles vaccine, which is available to patients over 65 without a prescription and is covered by Medicare. What luck that my store had a large senior population and we could capitalize on this opportunity to increase our profits in the pharmacy department.

After Zostavax came Pneumovax (the pneumonia vaccine). Over time, we were authorized to give every vaccine known to man. We were now vaccinating not only adults, but school aged children, who could have been getting their shots at the Health Department from a qualified nurse for 50 cents a shot.

While some pharmacists will dismiss my comments as the blatherings of a burned out old lady, they are missing the point. (This infighting, incidentally, is the reason pharmacists can't band together as a group and make a stand for our profession).

I am not averse to providing clinical services, in fact I would welcome the opportunity, but I do not agree with mass indoctrination of a whole class of professionals who did not originally go to school to give vaccines or prick fingers or, for that matter, touch patients.

To force needle phobic, blood averse individuals to perform tasks traditionally performed by nurses, infers a lack of respect and a blatant disregard for our profession and the professions of other members of the healthcare team.

Furthermore, I know myself, and the reason I did not go into a profession that required me to deal with life or death emergencies has everything to do with the fact that my mind goes blank and my hands shake when I have to perform a task under duress. Yet, in the event of an anaphylactic reaction to a vaccine, I would have been required to administer an Epi Pen injection, make sure emergency services were requested, and possibly perform CPR on the patient. This was not what I signed on for when I went to pharmacy school.

Our clinical services should be concerned with medication safety, simplification and education on drug regimens, helping patients navigate between their primary care physician and specialists, easing the transitions (where many medication errors happen) in and out of the hospital to home or an assisted living facility or extended care facility, maximizing cost/benefit of drug therapy, and a whole host of other huge problems that affect the piece of the healthcare puzzle we are most qualified to provide.

I also take exception to the expectation that we provide clinical services in addition to our other duties, like filling prescriptions and counseling patients. To allow patients to just walk in with no appointment, any hour of the day or night to get a shot, health screening, blood pressure check, or brown bag medication review session, is ludicrous. It sets the pharmacist up for failure, and it inconveniences the patient and causes them to regard us as unreliable and incompetent.

One of the reasons we were selected to administer immunizations in the first place, all day, every day, without an appointment, was because there is always a pharmacist on duty somewhere, any hour of the day, any day of the week, weekends and holidays included. Oh, how convenient, and what a great boon for those too busy or forgetful to make an appointment at their doctor's office, or attend a sponsored flu shot clinic. Just pop right in, 3 o'clock in the afternoon, or 3 o'clock in the morning, it's no problem. We are here to serve.

In 2013, Kermit Crawford, Walgreen's president of pharmacy, health, and wellness, told Forbes:

"We hope to eventually have the ability to administer all CDC-recommended immunizations in all 50 states, and for pharmacists to be recognized as providers in order to be reimbursed for immunizations and other primary preventative healthcare services. By offering a full range of immunizations in states that allow, we're able to provide even greater convenience

and access to vaccines and other preventative health services at our community pharmacies." (Forbes 2013)

We are "the most accessible healthcare professionals" because, unlike other practice settings, our "office" does not have a receptionist (or a door) to control access to our services. This accessibility is not by choice, as we would prefer to engage with one patient at a time, instead of fielding queries on the fly regarding everything from "ain't 'ya got no more mandarin oranges in the back?" to "how long is this going to take and how much will it be?".

Unfortunately, the chains abuse our accessibility and our tendency to be a walking encyclopedia, expecting us to be a cashier, a pharmacy technician, a stocker, an information giver, and a salesperson, in addition to being a shot giver, a prescription filler, a medication therapy counselor, and a damn nice person (or else).

Imagine walking in to your doctor's office and straight into an exam room, expecting to be in and out within 15 minutes, insurance processed, prescriptions written, and copay paid. And imagine the doctor taking care of all of these tasks in full view of you and all of his other patients, no nurses, no receptionists, just 'ol doc doing it all.

In fact, apply this scenario to any other profession besides pharmacist. Lawyer, dentist, CPA, loan officer, chiropractor, veterinarian, personal trainer, massage therapist, iridologist, fortune teller, voodoo priestess, witch doctor, it makes no difference. Not one of these other professionals stands tits out to the public, awaiting their pleasure, ready to field whatever is thrown at them at a moment's notice, and expected to be fast, courteous, accurate, and extremely nice throughout the whole transaction.

To envision our whore in a similar scenario, she might as well be lying on a bed, legs spread, in the middle of the town square, ready to serve all comers (pun intended) at a moment's notice, fair game for any Tom, Dick and Susie to have their way with her (or him).

Too far? I have been accused of this on occasion. For a less raw discussion of the open pharmacy concept, read "Close the Pharmacy", written by an pharmacist who calls himself "The Cynical Pharmacist" (Drug Topics, The Cynical Pharmacist 2015). In a later chapter, we will discuss another reason this open pharmacy concept has become a problem. In the midst of the Opioid Epidemic, pharmacy robberies have increased dramatically, putting not only the pharmacy staff, but the other employees and the customers at grave risk. Low pharmacy counters and multiple open windows make access to the pharmacy department extremely easy, and the lack of central alarms and security on premises is particularly negligent, considering what is at stake.

CHAPTER 20

WHORING FOR DOLLARS

HEALTH SCREENING AND MTM

The insurance companies began to provide incentives for patients to show up to have basic screening tests run in 2010. That was the year Insurance providers started encouraging Employees with HSA accounts to get health screenings done. They were given extra money in their accounts for getting the screening done and getting the necessary forms filled out. Many employers conducted on site clinics for their employees, bringing in a team of nurses to man each station, generally cholesterol screening, blood glucose screening, blood pressure screening, and weight and body mass measurement in comparison to ideal weight.

Walgreens corporate took it upon themselves to throw our hats into the ring and add us to the list of providers of these screening tests, since we had our magic NPI numbers and all, and we had so much extra time on our hands. Shucks, we already had the cheesy card table and cheap plastic table cloth stained with coffee cup rings and blood. Oh, and the "privacy" screen, which provided no privacy and served only as a tripping hazard for the patients.

So, they rounded us up and made us go to the District Office to be trained in a 1 hour session to perform cholesterol screening. We had already been doing blood pressure checks on demand, with an automatic cuff, of course, and had pricked fingers for blood glucose testing events held in the store in the past. Plus, we picked up a super-duper scale that not only measured body weight, like they do, but could miraculously calculate the amount of skeletal muscle vs fat, just by having the patient grasp a metal bar hooked up to the scale.

The cholesterol testing involved stabbing the patient in the finger (you needed a lot of blood) and siphoning it up with a very thin glass capillary tube. If you did not fill the tube properly, and there were air bubbles in the tube, the test could not be run. When people are nervous, or when they have poor circulation, they do not bleed well from their fingers. If their hands are warm, they are relaxed, or if they are on blood thinners, they bleed like the proverbial stuck hog. Bleeders made it easy to get a sample for testing. They were also the reason the testing area often resembled a crime scene.

Besides the obvious, there is another reason these screenings should not be thrown in with the day to day duties of the pharmacist. As hard as it is to believe, patients want to talk to you during the testing, like a real human being. Stepping out from behind the counter transforms the pharmacist into friend instead of foe. This is the kind of relationship pharmacists lost when they became assembly line workers, and they crave it as much as the patients do. Too bad for both of them, because as they chat, the pharmacy department is exploding in the background, and the patients waiting on their prescriptions are shooting daggers at you with their eyes.

Yet another seeming boon for the profession turned into whore bait by corporate was the evolution of MTM services. Patients with Medicare D, and a smattering of other insurance plans, were allowed one "brown bag" session a year in a private meeting with a pharmacist to go over their medications.

MTM or Medication Therapy Management, was designed to help increase both efficiency and safety as well as reduce costs by allowing pharmacists to finally do what they had been trained to do. Once patients were signed up for MTM, the pharmacist could document and charge for every service or recommendation they performed, including everything from recommending a cough syrup to suggesting a vitamin supplement.

The billing was accomplished through a company, often Outcomes or Mirixa, who provided the billing templates and software. The pharmacist filled out the necessary forms and made a note in the patient's profile that tipped him off that this was a MTM patient, thus serving as a reminder to provide as many services as possible to this particular patient and bill for them.

This was not stated in so many words, but the implication was clear. As you can imagine, the paperwork involved in documenting these interactions is nightmarish and required more training sessions to successfully navigate than that required to become an immunizer.

While on the surface this looked like the start of the answer to our prayers regarding our long hoped- for transition into getting paid to perform clinical services, in reality, our corporate pimps turned it into just another day of whoring for us. We were all required by our employers to get NPI numbers, which are the numbers assigned to us so our bosses could charge for our services and pocket the revenue. We were supposed to bill for each and every interaction, at $20 a pop, which, of course, required documentation and billing in addition to the interaction itself, which we had no time or support for in the way of increased staff or anything else.

There was another bump in the road that came up after the NPI numbers were issued. I used to have a fairly scant presence on the internet, and I liked it that way. After I got my NPI number, when I Googled my name, lo and behold there were scores of internet hits with my name on them. So, in addition to getting my whore number, I no longer had the relative privacy I had previously enjoyed online, courtesy of my corporate pimp.

MTM could be a very good thing, in the hands of independent pharmacists. There is a need for someone to help patients navigate the healthcare system, particularly with regard to their medication. I believe pharmacists could fill that need by starting their own MTM practices. Pharmacists were entrepreneurs in the days before the chains crushed their profession and their souls. Perhaps it is time to rekindle that proud tradition and strike out on our own.

CHAPTER 21

ROBBERIES, THE NEW NORMAL

As I mentioned in an earlier chapter, pharmacists are sitting ducks for any robber who wants to rob the pharmacy. On any given day, and sometimes for 24 hours, the pharmacy department is wide open, the store is practically deserted due to payroll cuts, and the pharmacist is busy multitasking. Many chain stores are near a major highway, which adds to the "easy in, easy out" advantage of robbing these stores.

The security measures, such as they are, do not make the pharmacist, the employees, or the customers safer. Most of the cameras that are installed in the pharmacy department are designed to catch drug diversion by employees. The one camera in the pharmacy that is trained on the counter, does show the potential robber that he is being filmed, because there is a screen mounted above the prescription pickup bins that shows him what the camera is picking up.

Of course, most robbers wear black hoodies and ski masks, so identification is somewhat difficult. At least the cameras are digital now, since, in the past, the managers would often forget to change the tapes and the camera would not capture the robbery. At any rate, this camera, with its "We're recording this robbery" display is supposed to be a deterrent to would be robbers. It's not.

The pharmacist does not have a "panic button" like a bank teller has. We used to have walkie talkies from Radio Shack at some of the stores for a while, but corporate got tired of buying batteries, I guess, so they did away with them. The things were attached with Velcro to the narcotic safe, and the idea was to press a button on the device which notified the manager, who hopefully had their device on them, that a robbery was in progress and to call the police. Like as not, though, the manager would come strolling back to the counter and say something like "did you mean to page me? That wasn't real, was it?" Well, if it was, you just got me shot. Be Well.

The next, greatest, brilliant idea is timed delay safes. How this is supposed to deter or protect anybody is beyond me.

"Hey, if you want to shop around, it's gonna be a half hour before the safe opens. I'll just call the police while you are not looking. I apologize for the delay. Thank you for your patience."

Right. In reality, according to pharmacists who have this system, the robber just hangs around until the safe can be opened. Nobody is calling the cops when you have a gun pointed at your head. I wonder which executive at the home office wants to stand there crapping his pants for a half hour until the damn safe opens.

Some pharmacists have purchased bullet proof vests, to the tune of around $600. My helpful question to one pharmacist who purchased and wore just such a hot, restrictive device every time he worked the night shift?

"What happens if they shoot you in the head?"

Some pharmacists break the "non-escalation" policy by carrying a concealed firearm. If it becomes necessary to use the weapon, they may save the customers, the employees, and themselves from harm or death, but the company will fire them, and so far the courts have backed up the corporations in such cases. (Drug Topics 2014)

Indiana used to be number 1 in the nation for pharmacy robberies. The latest report says we are now number 2. Every so often, some publication or other publishes a list of the states and how many pharmacies are robbed every year. If someone gets hurt or killed, the robbery is headline news for a couple of days at most. When I went to pharmacy school, robberies were rare. Now, they are an almost daily occurrence and nobody seems to see this as a significant problem. (Pharmacy Times 2017)

As if being robbed wasn't traumatic enough, the cost of the drugs lost in the robbery are listed as "shrink", so the $6000 or more in lost inventory counts against the store in terms of performance, and affects the bonus and pay scale for the store's employees when this line item comes up in their annual review.

One unexpected, but on the other hand should have been expected, result of the explosion of pharmacy robberies, was that, unlike in the beginning, where getting robbed would get you at least the afternoon off to calm down and get your shit together, current management thinking is that there is no need for the pharmacist or other employees to be so wimpy.

Other pharmacists who have been robbed and not been hurt or rattled by the experience are similarly *unsympathetic.*
"Did you hear about Mary? She took the rest of the week off after she got robbed! Geez, what a slacker. When I got robbed, I didn't even go home. I just went right back to working!"

Yeah, well you're an idiot. Go brag about your work ethic to someone who cares.

According to the Parable of the Faithful Servant:
"To whomever much is given, of him will much be required; and to whom much was entrusted, of him more will be asked."
— Luke 12:35-48

Therefore, here stands the White Coated Marvel, hands on hips, lab coat blowing in the wind, open to whomever or whatever comes along. Much like the Andy Griffith Show episode "Sheriff Without a Gun" the pharmacist is apparently supposed to use his wits to deftly handle any robbery with aplomb and never even soil his smock (or his underwear). Trouble is, Andy wasn't the only thing standing between robber and $50,000 worth of narcotics when he put his gunless self on the line. If Miss Elly, the Lady Druggist, had a narcotic inventory like that of the average Walgreens or CVS pharmacist, you can bet your ass she would have been packin'.

CHAPTER 22

CROOKED IS AS CROOKED DOES

They say don't judge a book by its cover, but they also say that the test of character is how you conduct yourself when no one is watching. Well, read 'em and weep, because the major pharmacy retailers have been in their share of hot water over their business and ethical decisions, and it has cost them big money.

Not that they seem to care all that much. Caught with their hand in the cookie jar, they issue a statement of contrition, pay the fine, and go right back to business as usual. Where you or I would be put in jail, the people responsible for the companies committing these violations continue on with their lives as if nothing has happened.

This lack of accountability trickles down throughout the organization, defining the culture of the company from the top down. If deception and denial are the order of the day, how far do you think they will go to make a buck at your expense off the back of their employees? Pretty damn far if you consider the evidence against them.

In 2013, Walgreens was handed the largest fine in the history of the U.S. Controlled Substances Act, when it was discovered that it's Jupiter Florida distribution center had committed "an unprecedented number" of record-keeping and dispensing violations. As a result, powerful narcotics and controlled substances were allowed to reach the black market, circumventing the procedures and regulations designed to make distribution centers the "first line of defense" in the distribution chains.

The fine imposed by the DEA was $80 million. In typical Wag speak, Kermit Crawford, president of Walgreens' pharmacy, health, and wellness division, issued a statement that Walgreens had taken steps to overhaul its ordering systems and train the employees in the proper procedures for dispensing controlled substances. Update the software, retrain the employees. Same old song and dance put forth by the chains every single time. Admit culpability? Not on your life. (USA Today 2013).

A side note to this sordid tale involves the aforementioned Mr. Crawford. He was often the spokesperson for the company when it came to federal and state violations of laws affecting pharmacy. In the wake of the Walgreens Boots Alliance merger, Kermit Crawford "retired" from Walgreens at 55 in 2014, receiving a "retirement payment" of $3.3 million and unvested equity holdings worth nearly $7.2 million. He stayed on as a consultant for 1 year, and was paid $1.5 million for this work. It's hard to feel too sorry for a guy that gets "forced out" with such a generous severance package. (Crain's 2014)

In 2012 Wag was fined $7.9 million to settle allegations that it provided $25 gift cards to patients on Medicaid, Medicare, and Tricare when they transferred their prescriptions from another pharmacy.

While this tactic clearly violates federal law, it also sets a precedent and gives an incentive for patients to transfer their prescriptions multiple times in order to gain the system. This may be good for the customer's wallet in the short term, it could cost them in the long run in the form of medication errors. Despite the incentives chains provide for patients to switch pharmacies, it is still in the patients' best interest to stick with one pharmacy. When prescriptions are scattered all over town, the pharmacist does not have a complete picture of the patient's medication and cannot catch potentially significant drug interactions or dosing issues. (CNN 2012)

In 2017, Walgreens paid a $50 million dollar fine to the federal government and the states for enrolling people covered by Medicare, Medicaid, or Tricare (which covers U.S. Military personnel) in their Prescription Savings Club, despite the fact that Walgreens published its own literature about PSC that clearly states these customers were not eligible for the program. The federal anti-kickback statute prevents beneficiaries of government programs from receiving anything of value from retailers who are trying to gain their business. Walgreens admitted no wrong doing and paid the fine.

At store level, we checked patient profiles to make sure customers were not on a government program, but some slipped through. Chain wide, with techs being paid up to $5 for each enrollment, the incentive to ignore the federal mandates was apparently too tempting to pass up. (Chicago Tribune 2017)

CVS has had its share of fines as well. In 2016, CVS reached a $3.5M settlement with the federal government after pharmacists in Massachusetts and New Hampshire filled hundreds of forged prescriptions, failing to recognize them as fake and report them to authorities. (Boston Globe 2016)

In 2009, While CVS paid $2.25M to settle with the Department of Health and Human Services over violations of the HIPAA Privacy Rule, a similar suit against Walgreens dragged on for five years, then was quietly closed, with no judgement meted against the company. The violations of patient privacy occurred after unsecured dumpsters containing patient information were accessed by individuals who wanted to steal information on patients, whether out of spite, or for personal gain. (HHS.gov 2009)

The full list of violations and fines paid by the top 3 drugstores (CVS, Walgreens, and RiteAid) are too numerous to list. In the Appendix I have included a listing of the top 10 violations and penalties paid by these three companies since 2010. (Good Jobs First 2017)

These settlements are disturbing, because they demonstrate the lack of regard that retail chain pharmacies have for laws that govern their business practices. Their disregard for patient safety is even worse.

CHAPTER 23

PHARMACISTS IN THEIR OWN WORDS

PHARMACISTS SPEAK OUT

I've been speaking my piece about retail pharmacy for a few chapters now. In fact, I just wrote a whole book on the subject. In case you think I am biased, jaded, or just plain full of crap, I have devoted this last chapter to my colleagues, the men and women who serve you on a daily basis and who are privy to all of the things I have written about and more.

Pharmacists speak out loud and clear. Anonymously. On forums like Topix, Reddit, and Glassdoor, and on Facebook pages, websites, and blogs, the true thoughts and concerns of pharmacists, and sometimes technicians, and store managers, are aired. They are well aware that corporate monitors these sites, and they take care not to identify themselves.

Unless you have a friend or relative who is a pharmacist, it is unlikely that you know or understand what goes into filling a prescription or running a retail pharmacy operation. Like most things, the best way to learn about a subject is to go to the source and get the information straight from the horse's mouth.

In the pages that follow, you will read actual excerpts from articles, blog posts, emails, and threads written by pharmacists. While all of them address different issues in pharmacy practice in different voices and styles, the main theme, the source of frustration, is clear.

The person behind the words is a highly trained professional doomed to spinning his wheels in a corporate nightmare. Contrary to what he was taught, he is no more in control of what happens in his pharmacy than is the high school kid at the front register.

ON THE CURRENT STATE OF PHARMACY PRACTICE

"It is nothing short of disgusting that we have allowed these chains of Greedy, Corrupt, Corporate non-pharmacist Businessmen to take over the profession. It is now unrecognizable."

"Our profession has been hijacked by corporate interests (chains, wholesalers, etc.). The pharmacy schools have just become another feeding ground or front for these interests"

"Money .... always follow the money .... corporations are amoral .... appeal to ethics is a waste of time .... money is their god...you have to be able to hurt them economically to get their attention/obtain concessions .... pharmacists blew their opportunity to control their profession long ago."

"After 35 years in the profession, I just do not see any light at the end of the tunnel."

"Who wants to have to worry about hurting or killing someone due to work environment when one's intentions while attending pharmacy school was to be a help to people?"

"What's happened to pharmacists? Many, if not most of their professional prerogatives have been removed from their exclusive purview, and handed to mostly untrained, non-pharmacists, with a lick and a promise that pharmacists will be used to provide other services like clinical pharmacy, inoculations, and medication therapy management."

"It's sad, but the reality of retail is that you will be abused and burned out until you quit or get fired, to be replaced with a naïve new graduate. I tell all the pharmacy students I meet to do everything not to have to go into retail.

"Working with techs who really wanted to run the pharmacy and reporting to management anything you did out of the ordinary. Working with supervisors and DMs who only were concerned about the bottom line. Corporate policies that protected the company and to hell with the employee pharmacist. I could write a book about my career and how I always put the patient first and maintained my character and dignity regardless of what was happening in the company. Label me bruised after 30 years in retail pharmacy, but still proud to be a pharmacist."

"Retail's a total joke now. I first got worried when WAG (Walgreens) started making fresh graduates PICs (Pharmacists in Charge) in my district a few years ago. (The more ignorant the better, I guess). That was the beginning of the end. The customers would much prefer more experienced pharmacists to consult, but the customer is powerless these days, thanks to insurance companies, and chain pharmacy domination of the market."

"...giving away products that can only be obtained from a pharmacy (prostitution of our profession). I have NEVER gone in a store and been given anything free of charge, ANYTHING that is life- saving (metformin or glyburide) or important to my actual well- being."

You're a faceless cog in a computer controlled environment...you're not a person or human being...your employer resents having to hire a license and would like to be paying you $5 an hour. Just as the govt./politicians have nothing but contempt for their passive "stupid" (in their eyes) citizens/constituents, your employers have nothing but contempt for your malleability and lack of spine. This country and pharmacy did not get where it is overnight...it happened in steps. A bully will push harder and harder until you fight back. Pharmacists acquiesced and said/did nothing for decades as the abuse increased step by step...level by level. Their passivity, selfishness, and inability to live life by principle never ceases to amaze me…how low will they go??...they are a mystery. Without organization and a national guild…without putting the profession ahead of selfish interests they are doomed."

"I am a pharmacist for the biggest chain in America and have also been a pharmacy manager for this chain. Upper management has taken our needed tech hours and is constantly demanding more, to the point that each day's work goes unfinished. Thereby leading to punishment in the form of decreased bonuses and extra "punishment work!" Every day is a horrible day, as not a day goes by that we are not disrespected by patients as well as doctors."

"Bottom line…pharmacy is just a reflection of the total socio-economic system of the US…apathy, ignorance, and denial, plus a lack of an organized response for decades by the American public (same situation in pharmacy) has given us an oligarchy riddled with oligopolies."

"As the pharmacy manager with no authority to do anything except deal with a lot of crap, I despised having to call for the store manager when I had an over ring at the register. I was not allowed to have a key to take care of it myself. That it inconvenienced the customer didn't matter. The manager ("store director") called the shots. I despised having to do paperwork that didn't matter. I despised being micro managed by my supervisor. I despised having to ring up a cart full of junk when I had customers waiting for their prescription. Possibly the thing that bothered me most was when techs were allowed to fill prescriptions, yet I was responsible if they made a mistake and I didn't catch it. With techs assuming more responsibilities, I wonder what pharmacists will be needed for in the near future."

"All we want, as pharmacists, is a little more help. We are dealing with people's lives, not hamburgers that may or may not have pickles on them. This is how the big chains see things, they do not care. All they care about is the $$ sign."

"The path our company is going down is going to KILL patients. Cutting hours in the pharmacy and making sure cosmetics is manned. Seriously!!!! This company is a Pharmacy chain. We are known as the Pharmacy America Trusts, not the pharmacy that gets it done in 15 minutes. Technicians are the safety barrier that we use to focus our efforts on verifying prescriptions, counseling patients, and ensuring everything else is right. Instead they give us this stupid G2 scheduling that is always 2 weeks behind. Now we (pharmacists) have to focus on filling, running out and getting OTC products, entering refill requests, drive thru, etc. The new catch phrase is This is My Walgreens. Well my Walgreens cares about service, not speed, focuses on keeping employees happy, is honest about intentions and doesn't try and break the very backbone that keeps this company afloat. Keep your employees *safe and happy and I promise we will increase sales. As it is now, we are so stressed out that there is no way we will ever provide the customer service you demand. Does anybody else think it is crazy that we can take 30 minutes to do photos, but demand scripts in 15 minutes? Put Pharmacists back in charge of the Pharmacy. Someone with an MBA has no clue what it is like to hold 250-700 lives per day in their hands*

"*I have been "fired" several times during the past several years because of concern about my patients, including being written up for not answering the phone in 3 rings when I had no tech help, being spied on by technicians who insist they know more than you do, drug addicts who insist on getting their drug of choice filled early, throwing tantrums and reporting me to management. The chains took away our benches, so we need to stand all day because they do not want us to appear lazy, no lunch, no breaks. I am exhausted, sad, frustrated, and suffering from post- traumatic stress syndrome. I have never experienced any of this in my previous years of pharmacy. We are no longer in control but are responsible for mistakes."*

"*Pharmacy has become a profession of employees with doctorate degrees who are usually addressed by their first name."*

"*Since corporations value only money, any appeals to ethics or reason are a waste of time...you have to be able to hurt their wallets...you must be organized, have lawyers, and most importantly speak with one voice."*

"I think it would be great if the media would spend a week at a busy retail pharmacy and get footage of what the working conditions are really like. The average person has no idea what the pharmacy staff deals with on a daily basis. I'd also suggest they are not allowed to take breaks or lunches like the rest of us are not allowed either. No chairs either."

"The media and cameras aren't allowed inside the store. Wonder why?"

"I likened my big chain retail job to a dairy cow or race horse continuously being pushed beyond safe levels with no feedback (aside from missed metrics/you're failing) and constant threat of decreasing hours. We became interchangeable licenses with no regard for effort, capability, dedication, or customer appreciation. The technicians have it worse, because those who care and work hard end up feeling responsible for picking up the slack for the pharmacists under dangerous pressure and for those technicians who do what they can/feel like with no concept of urgency. Until every single one of us behind the counter stop attempting superhuman efforts to meet metrics/corporate pressures and start taking breaks, eating lunch, drinking water, and actually going to the bathroom, and refuse to multitask with a telephone

plastered to our ear the majority of the day, there will be no change in retail practice."

ON NON-PHARMACISTS CONTROLLING PHARMACY

Robert Mabee is a frequent contributor to Drug Topics magazine and a pharmacist with a unique vantage point when it comes to observing and evaluating the current state retail pharmacy practice. He is a pharmacist, has his own law practice, and has his MBA. Check out his article: "Is Corporate Pharmacy Shooting Itself in the Foot?" (Drug Topics, November 10, 2015):

"Corporate bean counters and accidental employees do not understand the profession of pharmacy and the importance of pharmacy services. These non-pharmacists have tried to boost sales by cutting costs and reducing services necessary for patient welfare. Their goal is to sell larger quantities of expensive medications to boost total sales and temporarily increase stock prices."

The perception that pharmacists are just expensive employees has led to a business model that seeks to minimize the number of pharmacists needed to fill any given volume of prescriptions. This perception fails to recognize the opposing view and goal held by third-party payers regarding delivery of healthcare goods and services." (Robert Mabee n.d.)

AN ONLINE DISCUSSION ABOUT METRICS
From forums/studentdoctor.net:

"For those of us who work for CVS, how the heck do you get this metric up? Anything below a 5 destroys you. You can get 4 surveys of 5's each, then get one with a 3 or 4, and your MTD goes to an 80 automatically just from 1 survey. I know there are stores that just keep some receipts and give them to friends to do the survey. I don't think it is a good idea. But the way cvs emphasizes the metrics is that they basically want you to cheat to get the numbers up. That is what matters to them. As long as your numbers are up, you are fine. The end justifies the means. It is ridiculous how they are big on some random stupid metrics. Most people who work for cvs cheat to get the numbers up, it can be that they enroll everyone on ready fill, and so on......"

"You work at very busy stores that have technicians at every workstation. have you worked alone or with one tech for extended periods? I worked at a semi-busy CVS not too long ago and I had almost a tech at every workstation, it wasn't bad at all. when I floated to other CVS, that's when all hell broke loose. 90% of the CVS I floated to had little to no help. if there was help, it was a newly hired tech that was more of a hindrance. I quit right around the time they were transitioning to "my dashboard". Now, I'm at a national grocery pharmacy that gives me 4 FT + 2 PT techs DAILY. guess what? I don't need some survey to tell me I'm

providing good customer service or not. I will gladly provide top-notch service on top of MTM, immunizations, cholesterol screening and whatever they want me to do. why? because they give me ample help. I have floated at well over 30 stores and always have had ample help. can't say the same for CVS."

ON THE ROLE OF THE BOARD OF PHARMACY

"I would suggest the Board of Pharmacy may be the weakest link in any aspirations for pharmacy to lift itself above this seemingly impenetrable impasse. The profession is making remarkable inroads in gaining recognition for its clinical impact on patient care. But somehow, Pharmacy's hold on the thunder is short lived."

"Med errors are supposed to be up 455%...but no one cares-even the BOP's...but they are stacked with the same corporate pharmacists (non- practicing, of course) that are behind all the other problems."

ON THE ROLE OF THE FDA

"The FDA is responsible for ensuring prescription drugs are prescription-safe and therapeutically beneficial. However, they accept studies of the new drug effectiveness compared to a placebo. They do not test the new drug qualities against existing drugs, brand or generic. New drugs are not necessarily better or safer drugs, but are more costly"

ON WRONGFUL TERMINATION AND AGE DISCRIMINATION

"I was fired this year for a completely arbitrary reason, after being undermined by my head tech and store manager. Of course, I had no legal recourse because I work in an at-will state."

"I was terminated for misconduct two months ago. I had worked for the chain for seven years. I have applied to more than 20 jobs and have stopped looking for work. I am 62 years old and thankful that I could save enough for retirement".

"After 17 years of service, I also was unjustly terminated. I have since been able to secure another job another job. Age bias (25 yr veteran) or blackball? I have no idea. Terminated after 2 years of harassment from a non-Rph Market Manager that couldn't find any justified reason to fire me...and went to extreme lengths to try."

"I also read about the pharmacist who was marked for firing. This happened a lot in the chains, once they got 19 years in and received retirement benefits at 20 years, they were pushed out the door. I hired a couple of these people. Amazing what the chains can get away with"

"I have been the target of absolutely frivolous lawsuits, overly ambitious supervisors who have used trumped up incidents *to further their own careers, as well as being persecuted by countless techs who graduated from Mean Girls University Suma Cum Laude!! After nearly 8 years, I have had my fill. I now feel as if every single thing I do, or don't do as promptly as they would like, is being documented and tallied nine ways to Sunday, until they feel they have enough to terminate me, as I'm a female of a certain age."*

"I was an older pharmacist. I kept getting put into the worst pharmacy, and every time I built it up, they gave it to a guy. They would not give me a store near my home despite my seniority. They often gave it to a new graduate. They did it to several friends of mine that were older as well and had been with the company 35+ years. They forced them out before 65 yo."

"I was one of those do everything for the company guys. I worked for Safeway for 18 years and did everything I was told. Then Walgreens fiasco occurred, and all of a sudden we went from 1900 scripts to 3200 scripts in a matter of 4 weeks. I was the scapegoat as manager and got written up and transferred out. 6 months later they fired me."

"What is going on with the 3 letter chain? I left about a year ago, but my colleagues are basically being picked off one by one, some fired, some written up and basically forced to quit, it's very upsetting to hear!! Is this happening all over? When I left we had a new Rx supervisor who was horrible. I'm not sure if they are trying to get rid of older people who are making more money to put in new grads. I am just curious if this is happening all over, or if this guy is just an extra- large piece of work."

"They were after me for several years. Well not those places but still. And now I have an age discrimination case against them. Wish I really thought I would win. But I am sure they have some type of trick for that."

Jim Plagakis Rph posted the following on his blog on July 27, 2017. It supports the long- held intuition of legacy pharmacists that we are being unfairly targeted for elimination by our employers:

"It Is Official. CVS has issued verbal orders to middle management. "Get Rid Of Older Pharmacists and HIRE CHEAPER Robo-Dispensers". I received multiple phone calls over a period of 3 months from CVS pharmacists and one middle manager. They all told the same story. CVS is finding ways to fire older, veteran legacy pharmacists. These are 20 year, 30 year CVS employees. They are paid top rate. They have full benefits and all of them have 6 weeks of vacation annually. They have been in the same store for years Most of them Pharmacy Manager To. a person, the pharmacists who are already gone report that their replacements are children who got their Pharm D at one of *the for-profit NAPLEX preparation schools such as TOURO in Vallejo, California. None of these poor kids knows anything about compounding. They are completely OTC-ignorant. Pharmacy to these children is simple. They do what CVS tells them to do, Basically, make the Performance Metrics clock happy. Depending on the area of the U. S.A. their starting wage may be substantially less than what the poor !*@! (legacy pharmacist) makes."*

ON INSURANCE COMPANIES AND PBMS

"For over 36 years, I have had seminars on cardiac, blood pressure, tons of diabetic testing and brown bag sessions, etc. Now I am informed I am supposed to do more work for free to increase star ratings for insurance companies that have bullied me and paid me less every year."

"We have allowed the PBM middleman to abuse us and steal our business. I have complained to everyone I can think of, but the situation is very depressing. I think the worst thing that ever happened to our profession was chain stores and not because they are chains, but because the pharmacists are not owners, just employees. An owner would never "negotiate" some of the terrible contracts that are offered, while chains will. The chain works for its stockholders and I have no problem with this, but they also work for their patients, and we have let PBMs and insurance

intrude on the doctor-pharmacist-patient relationship with these middlemen even telling what drugs you can and cannot use."

"I have been a pharmacist for over 20 years, but now I am trying everything in my power to get out. I am/was a retail pharmacist, and I feel that my job has changed from helping people, the public, and patient education into trying to do anything to make a profit...like flog vaccinations. But the big bosses don't have a choice because they can't make a dime since the insurance companies refuse to pay, and then they turn around and take bad the rest of the money from audits."

"The Pharmacist is a distribution clerk. Gone is the very personal intervention with patients and their medical questions and concerns. 'Move 'em out, keep the prices low.' And the public will be forced to accept it, because the small independent is being forced out of business by insurance companies that are very much part of the problem."

"As you are probably aware, the PBM industry has been targeting independents for more than a decade, but now through their lobbying arm the Pharmacy Care Management Association, they are attacking our profession as a whole: http://www.affordablepharmacyaction.com/latest post/pharmacists-salaries-are-more-than-double-national-average/

ON ORGANIZING FOR CHANGE:

"It is only through public awareness can we hope to bring some form of change. It is the people at the bottom taking all of the abuse for the situation created by the corporations. Maybe if the public knew what was happening, they would be more tolerant of those at the front lines!!!

"I told my coworkers that I wished we didn't like each other so much, because it would have made it easier to let it fail. As it was, we each pushed ourselves harder so we didn't fail our coworkers in the trenches after us or with us."

"I was a pharmacy practice rebel all of my working career. For example, I even tried to organize pharmacists and start a professional "brotherhood" back in the 1970's. At first, I had a lot of support. Then guess what happened. Yup! Out the door by myself."

"I would love to start my own organization that represents pharmacists' interests but do not know where or how to start. APhA, NACDS, and the others do not do enough for us. State Boards do not do anything for pharmacists."

" I'm happy to report that I just joined TPA (The Pharmacy Alliance). I have reservations and doubts about regaining all that's been usurped by those who don't have healthcare, integrity,

mutual respect, and other principles as their guiding force or motivation. But, I've seen and been at the center of the progressive decline of workplace conditions and the management/micromanagement by those who have no business or qualifications to manage pharmacists, so I figure this offers more than trying nothing at all."

"You cannot survive on having your own business unless you figure out your niche, and still it's not easy, and you don't want to work for the chains because they abuse you to no end. We need to band together and make our voice heard. We are the one profession that does not stand up for ourselves, and that is why we constantly get kicked in the gut."

"I am frustrated that I didn't pitch a fit much sooner, but when you're getting your backside kicked so hard on a daily basis that you don't have time to go to the bathroom, It's hard to find time to plot a revolt."

ABOUT UNIONIZATION:

"We've been sold out by our schools, societies, and representatives. What we need are laws. Laws against monopolies, PBM abuse, regulatory abuse, etc. Unions will not solve problems; they will only create new ones. (Drug Topics 2015)

"We do keep management in line. They are always nervous that we will all walk out and go to the press with our stories. We, in turn, want to keep our jobs and serving patients. We negotiate at the table. Being a leader requires sacrifice. Management does treat you differently because of it. It can cost you money. But the sacrifice is worth it when it comes to saving the profession."

"I have been saying for years that we should unionize, to horrified looks. 'But we're professionals!' So are MD's and RN's and NP's and PA's who have what amounts to unions, and they have political clout. Pharmacists literally hundreds of little societies that have little clout. Now we are paying for that with jobs, salaries, and benefits. Current pharmacists will not benefit from unions, but maybe the younger ones will."

MCPHARMACY A RECIPE FOR DISASTER AND TRAGEDY!

(AN ARTICLE WRITTEN BY A 14 YEAR VETERAN OF CVS)

"Based on my 14 years experience as a pharmacist at CVS, I have concerns about the company's business model.

When there is a miss fill in the pharmacy, the first thing every patient wants to know is how could this have happened. If you look at the business model of the way chain pharmacies are now structured, it is easy to understand how Chain pharmacy has been headed in a dangerous direction for the last several years. When you start putting profit ahead of patient safety, you create an unsafe work environment with total disregard for public safety. Pharmacists today are doing the best they can under extreme pressure with the hope they do not harm a patient. With the understaffing and workload, pharmacists are doing the most with the least. The retail pharmacy chains look at the costs of this business model as a cost of doing business.

The average patient doesn't realize how physically/mentally depleted the average chain pharmacy's staff is now and all the non- pharmacist requirements pharmacists are being required to perform with most being simultaneously timed. Large pharmacy chains have only one goal- to maximize profits even if it means cutting corners on patient safety. Speed, metrics, and inadequate staffing all contribute to an unsafe dispensing environment no matter how many policies and procedures the company says they have in place. No matter how much technology *has been put in place, technology can only improve the efficiency of the prescription department so much. Short staffing and poor working conditions are pushing todays pharmacist and technicians to their absolute limits. Our job as pharmacists is to pump out as many prescriptions as possible with the least amount of help, while always multitasking to limit overhead. Also, many pharmacists are working long shifts without any kind of scheduled legitimate break to rest and maybe eat something. Whether a pharmacy is slow or busy, being understaffed and overworked with no break can lead to PREVENTABLE errors. However, pharmacists are professionals and not protected by many labor laws.*

Big chains could desaturate the market by hiring more pharmacist per prescription volume to alleviate the unsafe working conditions of the chain pharmacy. Instead, they focus on the number of scripts actually rung up through the register, rather than the total scripts filled by the pharmacy that week, and if that number doesn't equal budget, they will once again cut the pharmacy hours. They want you to have excellent customer service numbers with only a skeleton crew. Short staffing also prohibits time for the pharmacist to perform mandatory counseling which has been in effect since 1990 where many mistakes are caught before any harm is done.

The Pharmacy Benefits Managers (PBMs) have contributed largely to the understaffing issues. Before the PBMs, we were an all cash business-no price/profit controls-staffing levels were of little concern. PBM's provide a service not much different than

MC/VISA/AMEX. But unlike those cards, they control pricing, profits, and even limit where you can get your prescriptions filled, all of which can have an impact on pharmacy staffing levels In all, they take more money out of our healthcare system to support their cost/profit infrastructure, that could otherwise be devoted to patient care and safety.

Metrics need to be taken out of the pharmacy and patient safety should once again be brought front and center. The many metrics that supposedly are designed to measure customer care and satisfaction are in actuality used to increase profits at the expense of patient safety. Pharmacists are judged by the number of scripts they fill in an hour while multitasking. The phone lines are constantly ringing, a line at drive thru, drop off window, consultation window, e-scribes piling up, verification needing to be done, production needing to be done, calls to be made asking patients to refill their prescriptions (sales building in the guise of patient care), voice mail needing to be retrieved-all being simultaneously timed with the least amount of staff. There are so many metrics they are constantly scoring and adding, and as more production metrics are added, measuring production gets in the way of production itself.

Prescription volume and all this metric timing amounts to recklessness. To keep metrics in line, pharmacy department staff take short cuts which raise the potential for medication errors. Many retail chains see pharmacy as just a way to make money focusing on prescription volume, metrics, and squeezing every ounce of profit out of the pharmacy. Understaffed with too many metrics to meet and wanting you to go as fast as you can, filling and verifying scripts are contributing factors to PREVENTABLE errors. Along with this, scripts need to be pulled from waiting bins and backed out and returned to stock, cycle counts to be done, pending inventory to be ordered, stock received that day to be scanned in and out of stock scripts from the previous day filled. Workload planner needs to be accessed daily to check for any additional projects corporate had downloaded also to be done. It does not take a genius to figure out a person can only do so much in a given amount of time. We should be focusing on patients instead of trying to run like an assembly line out of control. Also, why are there no metrics for patient safety, patient care, or input accuracy? And when did the patient become viewed as just another customer and not a patient by corporate pharmacy?

The pharmacy department might as well be the grocery department in terms of respect for liability and patient safety. Walls are considered a barrier to the pharmacist and the patient and pharmacist function in a fish bowl environment with every part of it in full view and completely interruptible. Many times, pharmacists are interrupted by "Ahem-can you tell me where the toothpaste is , where the batteries are, why my prescription is taking so long" etc. further interrupting the prescription filling process and leading to an increased chance of error. Patients should be educated that it is for their safety and well-being that prescription filling be allowed a reasonable time without interruptions. Patients have been taught to want speed and accuracy and the option of counsel all on their demand. Having less interruptions and a better lay-out for privacy with sufficient staffing will lead to fewer mistakes that may harm patients.

When I was working for CVS, the stress and anxiety was insurmountable, and I was always fearful I was going to hurt someone trying to do all that was required of me in a given day. We averaged 228 scripts per day which equated to 3 minutes and 30 seconds per script to enter script, handle all insurance rejections, check for interactions and verify script, all while simultaneously doing the daily tasks on a skeleton crew. Imagine trying to keep up that pace for 14 hours with no break or food. A tired pharmacist is a dangerous pharmacist.

I guess for corporate pharmacy the important thing is that stock is up, profits are up, and the shareholders are happy. Please help educate the public to the reality of what is going on behind the counter. Then and only the, we can hopefully strive to make change and prevent PREVENTABLE errors from happening! Please share this with everyone so the public becomes aware of the dangerous working conditions!

A LETTER SENT TO 51 BOARDS OF PHARMACY

In January of 2012, Pharmacist activist Steve Ariens, PD, the National Public Relations Director for The Pharmacy Alliance, sent the following email to 51 state boards of pharmacy. As far as he could tell, he later reported on his website pharmaciststeve.com, none of the boards even acknowledged receiving the emails, let alone bothered to draft a response.

He finally did get a response from the Wyoming Board of Pharmacy, which I have included after Steve's letter:

Dear Pharmacy Board: Jan 12, 2012

We, at The Pharmacy Alliance, are concerned about the typical work environment of our colleagues and the patients that are being harmed because of errors resulting from such environments.

While we understand that most boards decline to address prescription volume and staffing man hours, we are concerned no board has addressed arbitrary time production metrics that are widely being forced on Rx dept staff. Study after study, involving many professions and industries, demonstrates a person working more than 8-10 hrs, particularly without breaks, becomes both less efficient and more prone to errors. Recently the Joint Commission published results of such a study
http://www.jointcommission.org/sea_issue_48/

We respectively request that each state Board of Pharmacy, place on their next agenda and discuss the implementation of mandates that will address these system- induced errors. With a reported 100,000 people dying from medical mistakes and 1.5 million being harmed from medication errors. We think that it is time to help prevent the next "Eric Cropp incident".

In our opinion, some of the health and safety issues that need to be addressed:

1. Prohibit any Rx ready in minutes guarantee or advertisement that promotes how fast Rxs can/will be filled.

2. Limit the number of hours a RPh can work in a given day to no more than 10 hrs, including breaks.

3. Mandatory 30 minutes meal break for RPh scheduled working => 6 hrs. If pharmacy is being staffed by a single RPh, require mandatory closing of Rx dept.

4. Drive Thru windows are to be closed when there is no tech support in the Rx dept.

5. Eliminate any/all corporate mandatory Rx or vaccination production metrics or quotas.

6. Other timed metrics (answering phone, drive thru, cash register) can only be imposed on ancillary/tech staff, not Pharmacists

7. Mandate that any settlement with a patient for medication error that involves a settlement, greater than the cost of the medication(s), be reported to the board.

8. Pharmacies will report these errors noting chain, store, Rph.

Any chain, store or RPh that demonstrates annual error rates in the top 25 percentile ... will have to submit to the board, a written plan, how CQI is being implemented/improved to reduce errors.

9. Any non-Pharmacist employee, of the permit holder, that attempts to influence the professional decision of a Pharmacist can be charged with practicing pharmacy without a license and/or permit holder fined for allowing such behavior, or both.

We would appreciate a response to our request, at your earliest convenience

Sincerely,

Steve Ariens, P.D.

THE WYOMING BOP'S RESPONSE TO STEVE'S LETTER

The response Steve received from the Wyoming Board of Pharmacy illustrates my point that government officials do not care about the public's safety, the health and safety of the pharmacist, or the proper practice of pharmacy, which they know nothing and care nothing about. This is a prime example of why the healthcare system is broken.

4/4/12

Mary K, Walker, R.Ph. Executive

Steve Ariens, P.D.

National Public Relations Director, Pharmacy Alliance

The Wyoming State Board of Pharmacy met on March 20-21, 2012 and reviewed your letter of January 12, 2012. They discussed the various suggestions for medication safety in the workplace of a retail pharmacy.

The board appreciates the efforts of your group to enhance patient care by improving work conditions.

In 2011 revisions to the Rules and Regulations, Wyoming Pharmacy Act, were proposed and approved by the board after a public hearing. A new section requiring mandatory breaks if a pharmacist worked six hours or longer was approved after some heated discussion. The rules package was sent to Governor Matt Mead but that particular section was struck from his approval. He stated that the board did not have the authority to mandate such working conditions.

The Wyoming Pharmacy Association conducted a survey through their website and collected information about meal breaks and other concerns.

Sincerely,

Mary K. Walker Rph

Jim Plagakis Rph commented on the Wyoming board's response in a blog post on his website jimplagakis.com:

"If you have any doubts about Mead's political loyalties, go to You Tube and view his inaugural address. If you are an independent pharmacy owner in Wyoming and you voted for this guy, your vote was another nail in your coffin. Wyoming is the smallest state (population). The Board of Pharmacy did the right thing. They lived up to the mandate to protect the public and the governor killed their action with little examination. All he could see was that limiting pharmacists to 6 hours with no break could hurt the big companies. Too bad". (Plagakis 2012)

A LETTER SENT TO GREG WASSON, FORMER CEO OF WALGREENS

The following e-mail was sent company wide, posted anonymously by a Walgreens pharmacist in 2013. It is addressed to Greg Wasson, CEO of Walgreens at the time:

Mr. Wasson,

As one of your fellow pharmacists, a customer, and a shareholder, I am horrified by the direction Walgreens has taken under your poor leadership. When he opened his first store, Charles Walgreen announced,

"We believe in working, not waiting; in laughing, not weeping; in boosting, not knocking and in the pleasure of selling products."

That is no longer your philosophy. A good retail leader looks at both employees and customers and tries to make the partnership workable and profitable. Under your leadership, things have become progressively worse and there are disturbing internal issues threatening the integrity of my company. Your patients are not safe in your pharmacies. A five-year-old in Nashville was given the wrong medication in spite of the pharmacy manager earlier asking for more staffing to address the stress levels. Under your leadership, medication errors have killed four *patients and cost shareholders more than $61,000,000 in verdicts against you.*

Throughout it all, your staff is burned out and stretched to the limit except you and your board, sitting in comfortable chairs, calculating how many employees they can afford to lose or how many patients can leave or die before things get serious. Let me assure you that we cannot consistently, efficiently and effectively deliver prescriptions medications SAFELY under current conditions. And while your latest victim was curled on the floor of his shower, dying from a medication error, you rewarded yourself with a 36% raise. That 36% raise also comes on top of Walgreens losing Express Scripts, Anthem, Caremark, and soon Medco, and others, costing shareholders over $6,000,000,000 in business. You are sadly willing to kiss off over billions of dollars because other companies will not cater to you. What arrogance! In front of the cameras, you tell pharmacists that there is no quota, there is no pressure to rush through a prescription, but when the press leaves, the pressure comes out to up the volume. Dollars cannot get into the cash register fast enough to suit you, and there is absolutely no thought to staffing needs, employee hours, or patient safety. Medication decisions are not being made by pharmacists, they are being made by non-pharmacist financial bean-counters. They take raw data and decide that two minutes is a safe amount of time to fill a prescription from data entry to pulling the correct medication and counting the pills to pharmacist checking and counseling the patient.

You are a pharmacist. Can you even pretend that two minutes is adequate time? When was the last time you actually set foot in a pharmacy, let alone worked in one? You have traded in your lab coat for a three-piece suit, wiped the dust off your feet, and never looked back to see how the company functions or fails to function. Who are you serving? Are you serving the shareholders, who have suffered billions in lost business and wrongful death lawsuits? Are you serving the staff, who are burned out beyond functioning? Are you serving your customers, many who have survived medication errors and some who have not?

I met you once and I am sure you have no recollection of that meeting. I was totally unimpressed with your lack of leadership. I asked a simple question and you responded that you would have to get back to me. The same is true for company meetings. You insist upon questions beyond provided in writing ahead of time. Has anyone ever gotten a straight answer from you without your handlers cuing the teleprompter? And how does someone run a company with absolutely no knowledge of it?

Please do not try to pass this off with some pre-worded answer about rewiring for growth. Anyone in business knows that successful growth means more customers and more employees, not round after round of employee cuts and customers taking their no-longer-accepted insurance plans to your competition. The Pharmacy That America Trusts is quickly turning into The Pharmacy That America Avoids.

You have brought the Walgreen family name down and have a moral obligation to resign. You have cost people their jobs, and you have put customers at risk. Let someone lead the company who can bring employee morale to higher levels, provide courteous service to customers, and grow the business as Mr. Walgreen intended, treating customers with decency and fairness, not passing off a cut-rate job, and treating employees the way you would want to be treated.

Sincerely,
Someone Who Cares

CHAPTER 24

ASKING FOR YOUR HELP

As a pharmacist, I am supposed to be the one taking care of you, the patient. Now, dear reader, I am asking you to advocate for me and my colleagues so that we can do the job that we were trained to do.

Our job is to dispense medications and counsel patients on the uses and effects of these medications. It is our great desire to help you navigate the slippery slope between your family doctor and your specialists, help you straighten out your medications after a hospital or rehab stay, and intercede on your behalf by contacting the other healthcare professionals involved in your care if we deem it necessary. If we had the support staff, the resources, and the autonomy to practice as we wish, we could give our patients the benefit of our many years of training and our expertise.

On the following pages, I provide a sample letter that you as a patient and consumer can send to your state Board of Pharmacy, the NABP, your Attorney General, and your Governor. The contact information for each state is included for your convenience. There is also a sample letter to be sent to the CEOs of the chains, along with their contact information.

There are over 250,000 pharmacists in the United States. This is not a huge number, and we have nothing to offer in the way of large campaign contributions, influence, or power.

Unions have not helped, and pharmacists are reluctant to join, both out of fear of retaliation, and because of our obligation to the patients. Even with documentation and a clear violation of our legal rights, it is difficult to even find a law firm willing to represent us against a huge corporation like CVS or Walgreens.

Pharmacists are dedicated, hard-working, intelligent, giving, and exacting, sometimes to a fault. We care about you and your health. We can't stand it when we make even the slightest error, and we hate not being able to give 100% to our patients, because we can't or won't organize, take off the Golden Handcuffs, and combat the blatant abuse imposed by our employers.

We accomplish a lot with what we are given. What we cannot seem to do is to take a stand and risk giving up our jobs and the income that supports our families to fight against a huge corporation with deep pockets, armies of corporate lawyers, and the ear of every politician and Board of Pharmacy from sea to shining sea.

A LETTER TO THE STATE BOARD OF PHARMACY, NABP, ATTORNEY GENERAL, AND GOVERNOR

JOHN AND JANE DOE
ADDRESS
PHONE   Date:
EMAIL

DEAR XXXX

I am writing to you today to ask you to use the authority granted to you by law, which mandates that you address issues in the practice of pharmacy that concern the safety and welfare of the public.

The Mission Statement of the NABP, as well as similar statements posted by the individual State Boards of Pharmacy, clearly states that they have accepted the responsibility for keeping me, my family, and my community safe with regard to the practice of pharmacy and the handling and distribution of medication to the public.

NABP Mission Statement:

NABP is the independent, international, and impartial association that assists its member boards and jurisdictions for the purpose of protecting the public health.

I respectfully demand that you address the following issues which are currently putting myself, my family, and my community at risk for harm or death from medication errors:
1. Lack of adequate staff in pharmacy department to handle workload.
2. Lack of staff, time, and privacy to perform mandated counseling on medications.
3. Extended wait times and lack of access to the pharmacist due to inadequate staffing.
4. Violation of HIPAA laws and lack of privacy due to design of pharmacy department.

5. Unlawful authority of the Store Manager over the Pharmacist in Charge.
6. Use of metrics to induce the pharmacist to rush and take short cuts.
7. Lack of half hour meal breaks and fifteen minute breaks for pharmacists
8. Immunizations and health screenings being performed in full view of other patients
9. Immunizations and health screenings being performed when only one pharmacist is on duty.
10. Violation of the law requiring presence of pharmacist in the pharmacy at all times.
11. Requiring pharmacy staff to push flu shots and other promotions to meet quotas.

Please take steps to address and rectify these long standing and obvious issues affecting the practice of pharmacy, and assert your authority over these matters to protect my health and safety.

Sincerely

A LETTER TO THE EXECUTIVES OF CHAIN PHARMACIES

JOHN AND JANE DOE
ADDRESS
PHONE   Date:
EMAIL

DEAR XXXX

As a patient and consumer, I wish to file a complaint regarding the long wait times and general disorganization of your pharmacy departments. Your pharmacy departments are understaffed and, at times, chaotic. I often see the pharmacist working alone, or with minimal help.

I do not think that having a technician ask me if I have any questions for the pharmacist satisfies the intent and purpose of the OBRA '90 laws governing patient counseling. How do I know what questions to ask? Shouldn't the pharmacist tell me what I need to know as a matter of course?

I do not like being pressured to get a flu, shingles, or pneumonia shot, and I do not want to be asked about donating money to charity when I am trying to focus on my medication, how to use it, or how much it costs. Loyalty cards and other store centered promotions should be handled by the cashiers at the front of the store.

I do not like discussing my medication in a waiting room where other customers are present. Unfortunately, this is the only place I can discuss my medication, since the pharmacist cannot get out of the pharmacy long enough to meet with me privately. The current pharmacy model violates my HIPAA rights.

I have seen other patients getting flu shots behind a flimsy screen in full view of the other patients. Some of the patients have to lower their shirt over their shoulder, exposing themselves to all present. There should be a private room for immunizations and health screenings.

Please do not send a form letter or canned response and tell me that you are looking into the matter and have spoken with your pharmacists and technicians in an attempt to rectify this situation. Your company has been avoiding the issue of pharmacy staffing and patient safety for years. You are the ones who set sales goals and staffing, and you are the ones who can change these policies.

I am writing to my governor, the Board of pharmacy, and the Attorney General regarding this matter. I would appreciate a personal response. Better yet, clean up your act and give the patients you serve the consideration they deserve.

Sincerely,

A LETTER TO CONGRESS

JOHN AND JANE DOE
Date:
ADDRESS
PHONE   Date:
EMAIL

DEAR XXXX

I am writing to you today to express my concern about the dangers faced by patients like me who have their prescriptions filled at chain pharmacies.

CVS, Walgreens, Walmart, Rite Aid, and other drug chains are endangering the public by not having adequate staff in the pharmacy, and by cutting hours of support staff while at the same time increasing the responsibilities of the pharmacists. They have been allowed to do this for years, and yet, nothing has been done to correct these dangerous conditions. Fines and monetary penalties have done nothing to induce these huge corporations to change, and are viewed as a slap on the wrist and a cost of doing business.

I respectfully demand that you address the following issues which are currently putting myself, my family, and my community at risk for harm or death from medication errors:

1. Lack of adequate staff in pharmacy department to handle workload.
2. Lack of staff, time, and privacy to perform mandated counseling on medications.
3. Extended wait times and lack of access to the pharmacist due to inadequate staffing.
4. Violation of HIPAA laws and lack of privacy due to design of pharmacy department.
5. Unlawful authority of the Store Manager over the Pharmacist in Charge.
6. Use of metrics to induce the pharmacist to rush and take short cuts.

7. Lack of half hour meal breaks and fifteen minute breaks for pharmacists
8. Immunizations and health screenings being performed in full view of other patients
9. Immunizations and health screenings being performed when only one pharmacist is on duty
10. Violation of the law requiring presence of pharmacist in the pharmacy at all times.
11. Requiring pharmacy staff to push flu shots and other promotions to meet quotas.

Please take steps to address and rectify these long standing and obvious issues affecting the practice of pharmacy, and assert your authority over these matters to protect my health and safety.

Sincerely,

NABP CONTACT INFORMATION

NABP (NATIONAL ASSOCIATION OF BOARDS OF PHARMACY)
https://nabp.pharmacy/h

Hours: Monday to Friday, 9 AM to 5 PM Central Time
Phone: 1-847/391-4406
Fax: 1-847/375-1114
Email: help@nabp.pharmacy
Mailing Address:
NABP
1600 Feehanville Dr
Mount Prospect, IL 60056

Contact NABP's Executive Director/Secretary
Executive Director Carmine A. Catazone
Email: ExecOffice@nabp.pharmacy
Press Inquiries
Are you a member of the media? We'll do our best to get you the information you need by your deadline.
Phone: 1-847/391-4405

The National Association of Boards of Pharmacy: Supporting Its Member Boards of Pharmacy to Protect Public Health
Founded in 1904, the National Association of Boards of Pharmacy (NABP) aims to ensure the public's health and safety through its pharmacist license transfer and pharmacist competence assessment programs, as well as through its VIPPS, VAWD, and DMEPOS accreditation programs.

NABP's member boards of pharmacy are grouped into eight districts that include all 50 United States, the District of Columbia, Guam, Puerto Rico, the Virgin Islands, Australia, Bahamas, 10 Canadian provinces, and New Zealand. The Association is governed by its Executive Committee, whose officers and members are elected during the Association's Annual Meeting.

NABP Mission Statement

NABP is the independent, international, and impartial association that assists its member boards and jurisdictions for the purpose of protecting the public health.
Vision Statement
Innovating and collaborating today for a safer public health tomorrow.

STATE BOARDS OF PHARMACY
WEBSITES AND CONTACT INFORMATION

ALABAMA
http://www.albop.com
Office: 205/981-2280
Fax: 205/981-2330
Susan Alverson
Executive Secretary
111 Village St
Birmingham, AL 35242

ALASKA
https://www.commerce.alaska.gov/web/cbpl/ProfessionalLicensing/BoardofPharmacy.aspx
Office: 907/465-2550
Fax: 907/465-2974
Email: **license@alaska.gov**
Donna M. Bellino
Occupational Licensing Examiner
PO Box 110806
Juneau, AK 99811-0806

ARIZONA
https://pharmacy.az.gov/
Office: 602/771-2727
Fax: 602/771-2749
Kamlesh "Kam" Gandhi
Executive Director
PO Box 18520
Phoenix, AZ 85005-8520
Email: **KGandhi@azpharmacy.gov**

ARKANSAS
http://pharmacy.publishpath.com
Office: 501/682-0190
Fax: 501/682-0195
John Clay Kirtley
Executive Director
322 S Main St, Suite 600
Little Rock, AR 72201
Email: **John.Kirtley@arkansas.gov**

CALIFORNIA
https://www.pharmacy.ca.gov
Office: 916/574-7900
Fax: 916/574-8618
Virginia "Giny" Herold
Executive Officer
1625 N Market Blvd N219
Sacramento, CA 95834
Email: **virginia.herold@dca.ca.gov**

COLORADO
https://www.colorado.gov/pacific/dora/Pharmacy
Office: 303/894-7754
Fax: 303/894-7692
Wendy Anderson
Program Director
1560 Broadway, Suite 1350
Denver, CO 80202-5143
Email: **wendy.anderson@state.co.us**
Phone: 303/894-2819

CONNECTICUT
https://portal.ct.gov/DCP/Drug-Control-Division/Commission-of-Pharmacy/The-Commission-of-Pharmacy
Office: 860/713-6070
Fax: 860/706-1242
Heather Hoynes
Board Administrator
450 Columbus Blvd, Suite 901
Hartford, CT 06103
Email: **Heather.Hoynes@ct.gov**

DELAWARE
https://dpr.delaware.gov/boards/pharmacy/
Office: 302/744-4500
Fax: 302/739-2711
Email: **customerservice.dpr@state.de.us**
Division of Professional Regulation
Cannon Building, 861 Silver Lake Blvd, Suite 203
Dover, DE 19904

DISTRICT OF COLUMBIA
contact Information
https://dchealth.dc.gov
Office: 202/724-8800
Fax: 877/862-4252
Email: **shauna.white@dc.gov**
Shauna White
Executive Director
899 N Capitol St, NE, 2nd Floor
Washington, DC 20002

FLORIDA
https://floridaspharmacy.gov
Office: 850/245-4292
Fax: 850/413-6982
Email: **MQA_Pharmacy@doh.state.fl.us**
C. Erica White
Executive Director
4052 Bald Cypress Way, Bin #C04
Tallahassee, FL 32399-325

GEORGIA
https://gbp.georgia.gov
Office: 404/651-8000
Fax: 678/717-6694
Email: **tbattle@dch.ga.gov**
Tanja Battle
Executive Director
Georgia Department of Community Health
, 2 Peachtree St NW, 6th Floor
Atlanta, GA 30303

GUAM
http://www.dphss.guam.gov/content/contact-us
Office: 671/735-7412
Fax: 671/735-7413
Email: **marlene.carbullido@dphss.guam.gov**
Marlene Carbullido, MSN, RN
Acting Administrator
123 Chalan Kareta
Mangilao 96913

HAWAII
http://cca.hawaii.gov/pvl/boards/pharmacy/
Office: 808/586-2695
Fax: 808/586-2689
Email: **pharmacy@dcca.hawaii.gov**
Lee Ann Teshima
Executive Officer
PO Box 3469
Honolulu, HI 96801

IDAHO
https://bop.idaho.gov
Office: 208/334-2356
Fax: 208/334-3536
Email: **info@bop.idaho.gov**
Alex J. Adams, PharmD, MPh
Executive Director
PO Box 83720
Boise, ID 83720
Email: **alex.adams@bop.idaho.gov**

ILLINOIS
https://www.idfpr.com/profs/pharm.asp
Office: 800/560-6420
Fax: 217/782-7645
Robert Gerton
Pharmacy Board Liaison
320 W Washington, 3rd Floor
Springfield, IL 62786

INDIANA
https://www.in.gov/pla/pharmacy.htm
Office: 317/234-2067
Fax: 317/233-4236
Email: **pla4@pla.IN.gov**
Darren Covington
Director
402 W Washington St, Room W072
Indianapolis, IN 46204-2739

IOWA
https://pharmacy.iowa.gov
Office: 515-281-5944
Fax: 515/281-4609
Email: **Andrew.funk@iowa.gov**
Andrew Funk, PharmD
Executive Director
400 SW 8th St, Suite E
Des Moines, IA 50309-4688

KANSAS
http://www.pharmacy.ks.gov
Office: 785/296-4056
Fax: 785/296-8420
Email: **pharmacy@ks.gov**
Alexandra Blasi
Executive Secretary
800 SW Jackson, Ste 1414
Topeka, KS 66612

KENTUCKY
https://pharmacy.ky.gov/Pages/default.aspx
Office: 502/564-7910
Fax: 502/696-3806
Email: **pharmacy.board@ky.gov**
Steve Hart
Executive Director
State Office Building Annex, Ste 300, 125 Holmes St
Frankfort, KY 40601

LOUISIANA
http://www.pharmacy.la.gov
Office: 225/925-6496
Fax: 225/925-6499
Email: **info@pharmacy.la.gov**
Malcolm J. Broussard
Executive Director
3388 Brentwood Drive
Baton Rouge, LA 70809-1700

MAINE
https://www.maine.gov/pfr/professionallicensing/professions/pharmacy/
Office: 207/624-8620
Fax: 207/624-8666
Email: **pharmacy.board@maine.gov**
Geraldine L. "Jeri" Betts
Board Administrator
35 State House Station
Augusta, ME 04333

MARYLAND
https://health.maryland.gov/pharmacy/Pages/index.aspx
Office: 410/764-4755
Fax: 410/358-9512
Email: **dhmh.mdbop@maryland.gov**
Deena Speights-Napata
Executive Director
PO Box 1991
Baltimore, MD 21203

MASSACHUSETTS
https://www.mass.gov/orgs/board-of-registration-in-pharmacy
Office: 617/973-0800
Fax: 617/973-0983
Email: **Pharmacy.Admin@MassMail.State.MA.US**
David Sencabaugh
Executive Director
239 Causeway St. 5th Floor, Suite 500
Boston, MA 02114

MICHIGAN
https://www.michigan.gov/lara/0,4601,7-154-72600---,00.html
Office: 517/373-8068
Fax: 517/373-1044
Email: **BPLHelp@michigan.gov**
Bureau of Professional Licensing/Licensing Division
611 W Ottawa, 3rd Floor, PO Box 30670
Lansing, MI 48909-8170

MINNESOTA
https://mn.gov/boards/pharmacy/
Office: 651/201-2825
Fax: 612/617-2262
Email: **pharmacy.board@state.mn.us**
Cody C. Wiberg
Executive Director
2829 University Ave SE, Suite 530
Minneapolis, MN 55414-3251

MISSISSIPPI
http://www.mbp.ms.gov/Pages/default.aspx
Office: 601/899-8880
Fax: 601/899-8851
Email: **fgammill@mbp.state.ms.us**
Frank Gammill
Executive Director
Jackson, MS 39211

MISSOURI
https://www.pr.mo.gov/pharmacists.asp
Office: 573/751-0091
Fax: 573/526-3464
Email: **MissouriBOP@pr.mo.gov**
Kimberly Grinston
Executive Director
PO Box 625
Jefferson City, MO 65102

MONTANA
http://boards.bsd.dli.mt.gov/pha
Office: 406/841-2371
Fax: 406/841-2355
Email: **dlibsdpha@mt.gov**
Marcie Bough
Executive Director
PO Box 200513
Helena, MT 59620-0513

NEBRASKA
http://dhhs.ne.gov/publichealth/Pages/crl_crlindex.aspx
Office: 402/471-2118
Fax: 402/471-8614
Email: **kathie.lueke@nebraska.gov**
Kathie Lueke
Office Administrator
PO Box 94986
Lincoln, NE 68509-4986

NEVADA
http://bop.nv.gov
Office: 775/850-1440
Fax: 775/850-1444
Email: **pharmacy@pharmacy.nv.gov**
Larry L. Pinson
Executive Secretary
431 W Plumb Ln
Reno, NV 89509

NEW HAMPSHIRE
https://www.nh.gov/pharmacy
Office: 603/271-2350
Fax: 603/271-2856
Michael Bullek
Board Administrator/Chief of Compliance
121 S Fruit St, Suite 401
Concord, NH 03301-2412 Email:
michaelbullek@nh.gov

NEW JERSEY
https://www.njconsumeraffairs.gov/phar
Office: 973/504-6450
Fax: 973/504-6326
Email: **RubinaccioA@dca.lps.state.nj.us**
Anthony Rubinaccio
Executive Director
PO Box 45013
Newark, NJ 07101

NEW MEXICO
http://www.rld.state.nm.us/boards/Pharmacy.aspx
Office: 505/222-9830
Fax: 505/222-9845
Email: **Ben.Kesner@state.nm.us**
Ben Kesner
Executive Director/Secretary
5500 San Antonio Dr NE, Ste C
Albuquerque, NM 87109
Phone: 505/222-9838

NEW YORK
http://www.op.nysed.gov/prof/pharm/
Office: 518/474-3817 ext. 130
Fax: 518/473-6995
Email: **pharmbd@mail.nysed.gov**
Kimberly A. Leonard
Executive Secretary
89 Washington Ave, 2nd Floor W
Albany, NY 12234-1000

NORTH CAROLINA
http://www.ncbop.org
Office: 919/246-1050
Fax: 919/246-1056
Jack W. "Jay" Campbell IV
Executive Director
6015 Farrington Rd Suite 201
Chapel Hill, NC 27517
Email: **jcampbell@ncbop.org**

NORTH DAKOTA
https://www.nodakpharmacy.com
Office: 701/328-9535
Fax: 701/328-9536
Email: **mhardy@btinet.net**
Mark Hardy
Executive Director
1906 E Broadway Ave
Bismarck, ND 58501-1354

OHIO
https://www.pharmacy.ohio.gov
Office: 614/466-4143
Fax: 614/752-4836
Email: **exec@bop.ohio.gov**
Steven W Schierholt
Executive Director
77 S High St, Room 1702
Columbus, OH 43215-6126

OKLAHOMA
https://www.ok.gov/pharmacy/
Office: 405/521-3815
Fax: 405/521-3758
Email: **pharmacy pharmacy.ok.gov**
Chelsea Church
Executive Director
2920 N Lincoln Blvd, Ste A
Oklahoma City, OK 73105-3488

OREGON
https://www.oregon.gov/Pharmacy/pages/index.aspx
Office: 971/673-0001
Fax: 971/673-0002
Email: **pharmacy.board@state.or.us**
Marcus "Marc" Watt
Executive Director
800 NE Oregon St., Suite 150
Portland, OR 97232

PENNSYLVANIA
https://www.dos.pa.gov/ProfessionalLicensing/BoardsCommissions/Pharmacy/Pages/default.aspx#.VjO9WGeFO7M
Office: 717/783-7156
Fax: 717/787-7769
Email: **st-pharmacy@pa.gov**
Melanie Zimmerman
Executive Secretary
PO Box 2649
Harrisburg, PA 17105-2649

PUERTO RICO
https://nabp.pharmacy/boards-of-pharmacy/puerto-rico/
Office: 787/765-2929 Ext 6641
Email: **junta.farmacia@salud.pr.gov**
Agustín González-Rivera
Executive Director
Department of Health, Call Box 10200
Santurce 00908
Email: **mirizarry@salud.pr.gov**

RHODE ISLAND
http://health.ri.gov/licenses/detail.php?id=275/
Office: 401/222-2837
Fax: 401/222-2158
Peter Ragosta
Executive Director
3 Capitol Hill, Room 205
Providence, RI 02908-5097
Email: **Peter.Ragosta@health.ri.gov**

SOUTH CAROLINA
https://www.llr.sc.gov/pol/pharmacy/
Office: 803/896-4707
Fax: 803/896-4596
Lee Ann F. Bundrick
Administrator
Kingstree Bldg, 110 Centerview Dr.
Columbia, SC 29210
Email: **leeann.bundrick@llr.sc.gov**

SOUTH DAKOTA
http://doh.sd.gov/boards/pharmacy/
Office: 605/362-2737
Fax: 605/362-2738
Kari Shanard-Koenders
Executive Director
4001 W Valhalla Blvd, Ste 106
Sioux Falls, SD 57106
Email: **kari.shanard-koenders@state.sd.us**

TENNESSEE
https://www.tn.gov/health/topic/pharmacy-board
Office: 615/741-2718
Fax: 615/741-2722
Reginald "Reggie" Dilliard
Executive Director
665 Mainstream Dr
Nashville, TN 37243

TEXAS
https://www.pharmacy.texas.gov
Office: 512/305-8000
Fax: 512/305-8082
Gay Dodson
Executive Director/Secretary
333 Guadalupe, Ste 3-500
Austin, TX
78701
Email: **gay.dodson@pharmacy.texas.gov**

UTAH
https://dopl.utah.gov/pharm/index.html
Office: 801/530-6628
Fax: 801/530-6511
Dane Ishihara
Bureau Manager, Division of Occupational and Professional Licensing
PO Box 146741
Salt Lake City, UT 84114-6741
Email: **dishihara@utah.gov**

VERMONT
https://www.sec.state.vt.us/professional-regulation/list-of-professions/pharmacy.aspx
Office: 802/828-5032
Fax: 802/828-2465
Email: **aprille.morrison@sec.state.vt.us**
Robert Enos
Executive Officer
89 Main St, Third Floor
Montpelier, VT 05620-3402

VIRGIN ISLANDS
https://www.vi.gov/contact.html
Office: 340/718-1311 Ext 3647
Fax: 340/773-1376
Deborah Richardson-Peter, MPA
Director, Office of Professional Licensure and Health Planning
3500 Estate Richmond
Christiansted 00820-4370
Email: **deborah.richardson-peter@doh.vi.gov**

VIRGINIA
http://www.dhp.virginia.gov/pharmacy/
Office: 804/367-4456
Fax: 804/527-4472
Email: **pharmbd@dhp.virginia.gov**
Caroline Juran
Executive Director
Perimeter Center, 9960 Mayland Drive, Suite 300
Henrico, VA 23233-1463

WASHINGTON
https://www.doh.wa.gov/LicensesPermitsandCertificates/ProfessionsNewReneworUpdate/PharmacyCommission
Office: 360/236-4946 Fax: 360/236-2260
Email: **wspqac@doh.wa.gov**
Steve Saxe, RPh, FACHE
Executive Director
PO Box 47852
Olympia, WA 98501/Email: **Steven.Saxe@doh.wa.gov**

WEST VIRGINIA
https://www.wvbop.com
Office: 304/558-0558
Fax: 304/558-0474
Michael L. Goff
Acting Executive Director
2310 Kanawha Blvd E
Charleston, WV 25311
Email: **michael.l.goff@wv.gov**

WISCONSIN
https://dsps.wi.gov/pages/BoardsCouncils/Pharmacy/Default.aspx
Office: 608/266-2112
Fax: 608/267-0644
Email: **dsps@wisconsin.gov**
Dan Williams
Bureau Director
PO Box 8935
Madison, WI 53708-8935

WYOMING
http://pharmacyboard.wyo.gov
Office: 307/634-9636
Fax: 307/634-6335
Email: **BOP@wyo.gov**
Mary K. Walker
Executive Director
1712 Carey Ave, Suite 200
Cheyenne, WY 82002

INTERNATIONAL PHARMACY BOARDS

BAHAMAS PHARMACY COUNCIL
http://www.pharmacycouncil.net/home.php
Office: 242/326-5066
Fax: 242/322-3118
Email: **bahamas@pharmacycouncil.net**
Anne T. Vanria Rolle, PharmD, MHA, RPh
Registrar
#23 Capital House, Corner of Virginia & Augusta Sts
PO Box N-4460
NP

NEW ZEALAND PHARMACY COUNCIL
http://www.pharmacycouncil.org.nz
Office: 64 4 495 0330
Fax: 64 4 495 0331
Email: **enquiries@pharmacycouncil.org.nz**
Michael Pead
Chief Executive Officer
Level 5, 80 The Terrace
PO Box 25137
Wellington, 6146

ALBERTA COLLEGE OF PHARMACISTS
Contact Information
https://abpharmacy.ca/?redirect
Office: 780/990-0321
Fax: 780/990-0328
Gregory E. Eberhart
Registrar
1100-8215 112 St
Edmonton T6G 2C8
Email: **greg.eberhart@pharmacists.ab.ca**

BRITISH COLUMBIA COLLEGE OF PHARMACISTS
http://www.bcpharmacists.org
Office: 604/733-2440
Fax: 604/733-2493
Email: **info@bcpharmacists.org**
Bob Nakagawa
Registrar
200 - 1765 W 8th Ave
Vancouver V6J 5C6

MANITOBA COLLEGE OF PHARMACISTS
https://cphm.ca/index.html
Office: 204/233-1411
Fax: 204/237-3468
Email: **info@cphm.ca**
Susan Lessard-Friesen
Registrar
200 Tache Ave
Winnipeg R2H 1A7

NEW BRUNSWICK COLLEGE OF PHARMACISTS
https://www.nbpharmacists.ca/index.html
Office: 506/857-8957
Fax: 506/857-8838
Email: **info@nbpharmacists.ca**
Sam Lanctin
Registrar
1224 Mountain Rd, Unit 8
Moncton E1C 2T6

NEWFOUNDLAND AND LABRADOR PHARMACY BOARD
http://www.nlpb.ca
Office: 709/753-5877 or 877/453-5877
Fax: 709/753-8615
Email: **inforx@nlpb.ca**
Margot Priddle, RPh
Registrar
488 Water St
St John's A1E 1B3

NOVA SCOTIA COLLEGE OF PHARMACISTS
https://www.nspharmacists.ca
Office: 902/422-8528 ext 229
Fax: 902/422-0885
Email: **info@nspharmacists.ca**
Beverley Zwicker
Registrar
1559 Brunswick St, Ste 200
Halifax B3J 2G1

ONTARIO COLLEGE OF PHARMACISTS
http://www.ocpinfo.com
Office: 416/962-4861, ext 240
Fax: 416/847-8200
Email: **aresnick@ocpinfo.com**
483 Huron St.
Toronto M5R 2R4

PRINCE EDWARD ISLAND COLLEGE OF PHARMACISTS
https://www.pepharmacists.ca/index.html
Office: 902/628-3561
Fax: 902/628-6946
Email: **info@pepharmacists.ca**
Michelle Wyand
Registrar
375 Trans Canada Hwy, PO Box 208
Cornwall, PE
C0A 1H0

QUEBEC ORDER OF PHARMACISTS
https://www.opq.org
Office: 514/284-9588
Fax: 514/284-3420
Email: **ordrepharm@opq.org**
Manon Lambert
Registrar
266 rue Notre-Dame Ouest, Bureau 301
Montreal H2Y 1T6

SASKATCHEWAN COLLEGE OF PHARMACY PROFESSIONALS
https://saskpharm.ca/index.html
Office: 306/584-2292
Fax: 306/584-9695
Email: **info@saskpharm.ca**
Ray Joubert
Registrar
Suite 221A - 1900 Albert St

AUSTRALIA PHARMACY BOARD
Contact Information
https://www.pharmacyboard.gov.au
Joe Brizzi
Executive Officer
GPO Box 9958
Melbourne
VIC 3001
 Phone: 61 3 9275 9

STATE ATTORNEYS GENERAL CONTACT INFORMATION

Steve Marshall (R)
Alabama Attorney General
Appointed: February 2017
501 Washington Ave. P.O. Box 300152 Montgomery, AL 36130-0152
(334) 242-7300
http://www.ago.state.al.us/

Jahna Lindemuth
Alaska Attorney General
Appointed: August 2016
1031 W. 4th Avenue, Suite 200, Anchorage, AK 99501-1994
(907) 269-5602
http://www.law.state.ak.us/index.html

Talauega Eleasalo V. Ale
American Samoa Attorney General
Appointed: January 2014
American Samoa Gov't, Exec. Ofc. Bldg, Utulei, Territory of American Samoa, Pago Pago, AS 96799
(684) 633-4163

Mark Brnovich (R)
Arizona Attorney General
Elected: 2014
1275 W. Washington St., Phoenix, AZ 85007
(602) 542-4266
http://www.azag.gov/

Leslie Rutledge (R)
Arkansas Attorney General
Elected: 2014
323 Center St., Suite 200, Little Rock, AR 72201-2610
(800) 482-8982
http://www.ag.arkansas.gov

Xavier Becerra (D)
California Attorney General
Appointed: 2017
1300 I St., Ste. 1740, Sacramento, CA 95814
(916) 445-9555
http://ag.ca.gov/

Cynthia H. Coffman (R)
Colorado Attorney General
Elected: 2014
Ralph L. Carr Colorado Judicial Center 1300 Broadway, 10th Floor, Denver, CO 80203
(720) 508-6000
http://www.coloradoattorneygeneral.gov/

George Jepsen (D)
Connecticut Attorney General
Elected: 2010, 2014
55 Elm St., Hartford, CT 06106
(860) 808-5318
http://www.ct.gov/ag/

Karl A. Racine (D)
District of Columbia Attorney General
Elected: 2014
441 4th Street, NW, Suite 1100S, Washington, DC 20001
(202) 727-3400
http://oag.dc.gov/

Matthew Denn (D)
Delaware Attorney General
Elected: 2014
Carvel State Office Bldg., 820 N. French St., Wilmington, DE 19801
(302) 577-8338
http://attorneygeneral.delaware.gov/

Pam Bondi (R)
Florida Attorney General
Elected: 2010, 2014
The Capitol, PL 01, Tallahassee, FL 32399-1050
(850) 414-3300
http://myfloridalegal.com/

Chris Carr (R)
Georgia Attorney General
Appointed: 2016
40 Capitol Square, SW, Atlanta, GA 30334-1300
(404) 656-3300
http://law.ga.gov/

Elizabeth Barrett-Anderson
Guam Attorney General
Elected: 2014
Office of the Attorney General, ITC Building, 590 S. Marine Corps Dr, Ste. 706, Tamuning, Guam 96913
http://www.guamag.org/

Douglas S. Chin (D)
Hawaii Attorney General
Appointed: 2015
425 Queen St., Honolulu, HI 96813
(808) 586-1500
http://ag.hawaii.gov/

Lawrence Wasden (R)
Idaho Attorney General
Elected: 2002, 2006, 2010, 2014
700 W. Jefferson Street, Suite 210, P.O. Box 83720, Boise, ID 83720-1000
(208) 334-2400
http://www.ag.idaho.gov/

Lisa Madigan (D)
Illinois Attorney General
Elected: 2002, 2006, 2010, 2014
James R. Thompson Ctr., 100 W. Randolph St., Chicago, IL 60601
(312) 814-3000
http://illinoisattorneygeneral.gov/

Curtis T. Hill, Jr. (R)
Indiana Attorney General
Elected: 2016
Indiana Government Center South - 5th Floor, 302 West Washington Street, Indianapolis, IN 46204
(317) 232-6201
http://www.in.gov/attorneygeneral/

Tom Miller (D)
Iowa Attorney General
Elected: 1978, 1982, 1986, 1994, 1998, 2002, 2006, 2010, 2014
Hoover State Office Bldg., 1305 E. Walnut, Des Moines, IA 50319
(515) 281-5164
http://www.iowaattorneygeneral.gov

Derek Schmidt (R)
Kansas Attorney General
Elected: 2010, 2014
120 S.W. 10th Ave., 2nd Fl., Topeka, KS 66612-1597
(785) 296-2215
https://www.ag.ks.gov/

Andy Beshear (D)
Kentucky Attorney General
Elected: 2015
700 Capitol Avenue, Capitol Building, Suite 118, Frankfort, KY 40601
502-696-5300
http://ag.ky.gov/

Jeff Landry (R)
Louisiana Attorney General
Elected: 2015
P.O. Box 94095, Baton Rouge, LA 70804-4095
225-326-6000
http://www.ag.state.la.us/

Janet T. Mills (D)
Maine Attorney General
Appointed: 2008, 2012, 2014
State House Station 6, Augusta, ME 04333
(207) 626-8800
http://www.maine.gov/ag/

Brian Frosh (D)
Maryland Attorney General
Elected: 2014
200 St. Paul Place, Baltimore, MD 21202-2202
(410) 576-6300
http://www.marylandattorneygeneral.gov/

Maura Healey (D)
Massachusetts Attorney General
Elected: 2014
1 Ashburton Place, Boston, MA 02108-1698
(617) 727-2200
http://www.mass.gov/ago/

Bill Schuette (R)
Michigan Attorney General
Elected: 2010, 2014
P.O.Box 30212, 525 W. Ottawa St., Lansing, MI 48909-0212
(517) 373-1110
http://www.michigan.gov/ag

Lori Swanson (D)
Minnesota Attorney General
Elected: 2006, 2010, 2014
Suite 102, State Capital 75 Dr. Martin Luther King, Jr. Blvd.
Saint Paul, MN 55155
(651) 296-3353 or 1-800-657-3787 | TTY: (651) 297-7206 or 1-800-366-4812
http://www.ag.state.mn.us/

Jim Hood (D)
Mississippi Attorney General
Elected: 2003, 2007, 2011, 2015
Department of Justice, P.O. Box 220, Jackson, MS 39205
(601) 359-3680
http://www.ago.state.ms.us/

Joshua D. Hawley (R)
Missouri Attorney General
Elected: 2016
Supreme Ct. Bldg., 207 W. High St., Jefferson City, MO 65101
573-751-3321
http://ago.mo.gov/

Tim Fox (R)
Montana Attorney General
Elected: 2012
Justice Bldg., 215 N. Sanders, Helena, MT 59620-1401
(406) 444-2026
https://doj.mt.gov/

Doug Peterson (R)
Nebraska Attorney General
Elected: 2014
State Capitol, P.O.Box 98920, Lincoln, NE 68509-8920
(402) 471-2682
http://www.ago.ne.gov/

Adam Paul Laxalt (R)
Nevada Attorney General
Elected: 2014
Old Supreme Ct. Bldg., 100 N. Carson St., Carson City, NV 89701
(775) 684-1100
http://ag.nv.gov/

Gordon MacDonald (R)
New Hampshire Attorney General
Appointed: 2017
33 Capitol Street Concord, NH 03301
(603) 271-3658
https://www.doj.nh.gov/index.htm

Christopher S. Porrino
New Jersey Attorney General
Appointed: June 2016
Richard J. Hughes Justice Complex, 25 Market Street P.O. Box 080 Trenton, NJ 08625
(609) 292-8740
http://www.state.nj.us/lps/

Hector Balderas (D)
New Mexico Attorney General
Elected: 2014
P.O. Drawer 1508, Santa Fe, NM 87504-1508
(505) 490-4060

Eric Schneiderman (D)
New York Attorney General
Elected: 2010, 2014
Dept. of Law - The Capitol, 2nd fl., Albany, NY 12224
(518) 474-7330
http://www.ag.ny.gov/

Josh Stein (D)
North Carolina Attorney General
Elected: 2016
Dept. of Justice, P.O.Box 629, Raleigh, NC 27602-0629
(919) 716-6400
http://www.ncdoj.gov/

Wayne Stenehjem (R)
North Dakota Attorney General
Elected: 2000, 2004, 2006, 2010, 2014
State Capitol, 600 E. Boulevard Ave., Bismarck, ND 58505-0040
(701) 328-2210
http://www.ag.state.nd.us

Edward Manibusan
Northern Mariana Islands Attorney General
Elected: 2014
Administration Building, P.O. Box 10007, Saipan MP 96950-8907
(670) 664-2341

Mike DeWine (R)
Ohio Attorney General
Elected: 2010, 2014
State Office Tower, 30 E. Broad St., Columbus, OH 43266-0410
(614) 466-4320
http://www.ohioattorneygeneral.gov/

Mike Hunter (R)
Oklahoma Attorney General
Appointed: February 2017
313 NE 21st Street, Oklahoma City, OK 73105
(405) 521-3921
http://www.oag.state.ok.us/

Ellen F. Rosenblum (D)
Oregon Attorney General
Appointed June 2012, Elected: November 2012
Justice Bldg., 1162 Court St., NE, Salem, OR 97301
503-378-6002
http://www.doj.state.or.us/

Josh Shapiro (D)
Pennsylvania Attorney General
Elected: 2016
Pennsylvania Office of Attorney General, 16th Floor, Strawberry Square, Harrisburg, PA 17120
717-787-3391
https://www.attorneygeneral.gov/

Wanda Vàzquez Garced
Puerto Rico Attorney General
Appointed: January 2017
PO Box 902192, San Juan, PR, 00902-0192
787-721-2900
http://www.justicia.gobierno.pr/

Peter Kilmartin (D)
Rhode Island Attorney General
Elected: 2010, 2014
150 S. Main St., Providence, RI 02903
(401) 274-4400
www.riag.ri.gov

Alan Wilson (R)
South Carolina Attorney General
Elected: 2010, 2014
Rembert C. Dennis Office Bldg., P.O.Box 11549, Columbia, SC 29211-1549
(803) 734-3970
http://www.scattorneygeneral.org

Marty J. Jackley (R)
South Dakota Attorney General
Appointed: 2009, Elected: 2010, 2014
1302 East Highway 14, Suite 1, Pierre, SD 57501-8501
(605) 773-3215
http://atg.sd.gov/

Herbert H. Slatery, III (R)
Tennessee Attorney General
Appointed: October 1, 2014
425 5th Avenue North, Nashville, TN 37243
615-741-3491
http://www.tn.gov/attorneygeneral

Ken Paxton (R)
Texas Attorney General
Elected: 2014
Capitol Station, P.O.Box 12548, Austin, TX 78711-2548
(512) 463-2100
https://www.texasattorneygeneral.gov/

Sean Reyes (R)
Utah Attorney General
Elected: 2016, Special Election: 2014, Appointed: 2013:
State Capitol, Rm. 236, Salt Lake City, UT 84114-0810
(801) 538-9600
http://attorneygeneral.utah.gov/

TJ Donovan (D)
Vermont Attorney General
Elected: 2016
109 State St., Montpelier, VT 05609-1001
(802) 828-3173
http://www.atg.state.vt.us/

Claude E. Walker
Virgin Islands
34-38 Kronprindsens Gade, GERS Building, 2nd Floor, St. Thomas, Virgin Islands 00802
(340) 774-5666
http://usvidoj.codemeta.com/

Mark Herring (D)
Virginia Attorney General
Elected: 2013
202 North Ninth Street, Richmond, VA 23219
(804) 786-2071
http://www.oag.state.va.us/

Bob Ferguson (D)
Washington Attorney General
Elected: 2012
1125 Washington St. SE, PO Box 40100, Olympia, WA 98504-0100
(360) 753-6200
http://www.atg.wa.gov

Patrick Morrisey (R)
West Virginia Attorney General
Elected: 2012
State Capitol, 1900 Kanawha Blvd. , E., Charleston, WV 25305
(304) 558-2021
http://www.wvago.gov/

Brad Schimel (R)
Wisconsin Attorney General
Elected: 2014
Wisconsin Department of Justice, State Capitol, Room 114 East P. O. Box 7857, Madison, WI 53707-7857
(608) 266-1221
http://www.doj.state.wi.us

Peter K. Michael
Wyoming Attorney General
Appointed: July 2013
State Capitol Bldg., Cheyenne, WY 82002
(307) 777-7841
http://attorneygeneral.state.wy.us

GOVERNORS' CONTACT INFORMATION

Please note: NGA does not maintain a list of Governors' email addresses. We suggest you visit your Governor's website and follow the instructions there on how to contact him or her.

Alabama
Office of Governor Kay Ivey
State Capitol
600 Dexter Avenue
Montgomery, AL 36130-2751
Phone: 334/242-7100
Fax: 334/353-0004
https://governor.alabama.gov

Alaska
Office of Governor Bill Walker
State Capitol
P.O. Box 110001
Juneau, AK 99811-0001
Phone: 907/465-3500
Fax: 907/465-3532
https://gov.alaska.gov

American Samoa
Office of Governor Lolo Matalasi Moliga
Executive Office Building
Third Floor
Utulei, Pago Pago, AS 96799
Phone: 011/684/633-4116
Fax: 011/684/633-2269
https://www.americansamoa.gov/office-of-the-governor

Arizona
Office of Governor Doug Ducey
State Capitol
1700 West Washington
Phoenix, AZ 85007
Phone: 602/542-4331
Fax: 602/542-7601
https://azgovernor.gov

Arkansas
Office of Governor Asa Hutchinson
State Capitol
Room 250
Little Rock, AR 72201
Phone: 501/682-2345
Fax: 501/682-1382
https://governor.arkansas.gov/

California
Office of Governor Edmund Brown
State Capitol
Sute 1173
Sacramento, CA 95814
Phone: 916/445-2841
Fax: 916/558-3160
https://www.gov.ca.gov/

Colorado
Office of Governor John Hickenlooper
136 State Capitol
Denver, CO 80203-1792
Phone: 303/866-2471
Fax: 303/866-2003
https://www.colorado.gov/governor/

Connecticut
Office of Governor Dan Malloy
210 Capitol Avenue
Hartford, CT 06106
Phone: 800/406-1527
Fax: 860/524-7395
https://www.governor.ct.gov

Delaware
Office of Governor John Carney
Legislative Hall
Dover, DE 19901
Phone: 302/744-4101
Fax: 302/739-2775
https://governor.delaware.gov

Florida
Office of Governor Rick Scott
PL 05 The Capitol
400 South Monroe Street
Tallahassee, FL 32399-0001
Phone: 850/488-7146
Fax: 850/487-0801
https://www.flgov.com

Georgia
Office of Governor Nathan Deal
203 State Capitol
Atlanta, GA 30334
Phone: 404/656-1776
Fax: 404/657-7332
https://gov.georgia.gov

Guam
Office of Governor Eddie Calvo
Executive Chamber
P.O. Box 2950
Agana, GU 96932
Phone: 671/472-8931
Fax: 671/477-4826
http://governor.guam.gov

Hawaii
Office of Governor David Ige
Executive Chambers
State Capitol
Honolulu, HI 96813
Phone: 808/586-0034
Fax: 808/586-0006
http://governor.hawaii.gov

Idaho
Office of Governor C.L "Butch" Otter
700 West Jefferson
Second Floor
Boise, ID 83702
Phone: 208/334-2100
Fax: 208/334-2175
https://gov.idaho.gov

Illinois
Office of Governor Bruce Rauner
State Capitol
207 Statehouse
Springfield, IL 62706
Phone: 217/782-0244
Fax: 217/524-4049
https://www2.illinois.gov/gov/Pages/default.aspx

Indiana
Office of Governor Eric Holcomb
State House
Room 206
Indianapolis, IN 46204-2797
Phone: 317/232-4567
Fax: 317/232-3443
https://www.in.gov/gov/index.htm

Iowa
Office of Governor Kim Reynolds
State Capitol
Des Moines, IA 50319-0001
Phone: 515/ 281-5211
Fax: 515/281-6611
https://governor.iowa.gov

Kansas
Office of Governor Sam Brownback
Capitol
300 SW 10th Avenue, Suite 212S
Topeka, KS 66612-1590
Phone: 785/296-3232
Fax: 785/296-7973
https://governor.kansas.gov

Kentucky
Office of Governor Matt Bevin
700 Capitol Ave., Suite 100
Frankfort, KY 40601
Phone: 502/564-2611
Fax: 502/564-0437
http://governor.ky.gov

Louisiana
Office of Governor John Bel Edwards
P. O. Box 94004
Baton Rouge, LA 70804-9004
Phone: 225/342-7015
Fax: 225/342-7099
http://gov.louisiana.gov

Maine
Office of Governor Paul LePage
#1 State House Station
Augusta, ME 04333
Phone: 207/287-3531
Fax: 207/287-1034
ehttps://www.maine.gov/governor/lepage/

Maryland
Office of Governor Larry Hogan
State House
100 State Circle
Annapolis, MD 21401
Phone: 410/974-3901
Fax: 410/974-3275
http://governor.maryland.gov

Massachusetts
Office of Governor Charlie Baker
State House
Office of the Governor, Room 360
Boston, MA 02133
Phone: 617/725-4005
Fax: 617/727-9725
https://www.mass.gov/orgs/office-of-the-governor

Michigan
Office of Governor Rick Snyder
P.O. Box 30013
Lansing, MI 48909
Phone: 517/373-3400
Fax: 517/335-6863
https://www.michigan.gov/snyder/

Minnesota
Office of Governor Mark Dayton
130 State Capitol
75 Rev. Dr. Martin Luther King, Jr. Boulevard
St. Paul, MN 55155
Phone: 651/201-3400
Fax: 651/797-1850
https://mn.gov/governor/

Mississippi
Office of Governor Phil Bryant
P.O. Box 139
Jackson, MS 39205
Phone: 601/359-3150
Fax: 601/359-3741
http://www.governorbryant.ms.gov/Pages/default.aspx

Missouri
Office of Governor Eric Greitens
Capitol Building
Room 216, P.O. Box 720
Jefferson City, MO 65102
Phone: 573/751-3222
Fax: 573/526-3291
https://governor.mo.gov

Montana
Office of Governor Steve Bullock
State Capitol
Helena, MT 59620-0801
Phone: 406/444-3111
Fax: 406/444-5529
http://governor.mt.gov

Nebraska
Office of Governor Pete Ricketts
P.O. Box 94848
Lincoln, NE 68509-4848
Phone: 402/471-2244
Fax: 402/471-6031
https://governor.nebraska.gov

Nevada
Office of Governor Brian Sandoval
Capitol Building
Carson City, NV 89701
Phone: 775/684-5670
Fax: 775/684-5683
http://gov.nv.gov

New Hampshire
Office of Governor Chris Sununu
Office of the Governor
107 North Main Street, Room 208
Concord, NH 03301
Phone: 603/271-2121
Fax: 603/271-7640
https://www.governor.nh.gov

New Jersey
Office of Governor Chris Christie
The State House
P.O. Box 001
Trenton, NJ 08625
Phone: 609/292-6000
Fax: 609/292-3454
https://www.state.nj.us/governor/

New Mexico
Office of Governor Susana Martinez
State Capitol
Fourth Floor
Santa Fe, NM 87501
Phone: 505/476-2200
Fax: 505/476-2226
http://www.governor.state.nm.us

New York
Office of Governor Andrew Cuomo
State Capitol
Albany, NY 12224
Phone: 518/ 474-8390
ehttps://www.governor.ny.gov
North Carolina
Office of Governor Roy Cooper
Office of the Governor
20301 Mail Service Center
Raleigh, NC 27699-0301
Phone: 919/814-2000
Fax: 919/733-2120
https://governor.nc.gov
North Dakota
Office of Governor Doug Burgum
Dept. 101
600 E. Boulevard Ave.
Bismarck, ND 58505-0001
Phone: 701/328-2200
Fax: 701/328-2205
https://www.governor.nd.gov
Northern Mariana Islands
Office of Governor Ralph Deleon Guerrero Torres
Caller Box 10007
Saipan, MP 96950
Phone: 670/664-2280
Fax: 670/664-2211
https://gov.mp
Ohio
Office of Governor John Kasich
30th Floor
77 South High Street
Columbus, OH 43215
Phone: 614/466-3555
Fax: 614/466-9354
http://governor.ohio.gov

Oklahoma
Office of Governor Mary Fallin
Capitol Building
2300 Lincoln Blvd., Rm. 212
Oklahoma City, OK 73105
Phone: 405/ 521-2342
Fax: 405/521-3353
https://www.ok.gov/governor/
Oregon
Office of Governor Kate Brown
State Capitol, Room 160
900 Court St. N.
Salem, OR 97301
Phone: 503/378-4582
Fax: 503/378-8970
https://www.oregon.gov/gov/pages/index.aspx
Pennsylvania
Office of Governor Tom Wolf
Room 225
Main Capitol Building
Harrisburg, PA 17120
Phone: 717/787-2500
Fax: 717/772-8284
https://www.governor.pa.gov
Puerto Rico
Office of Governor Ricardo Rosselló
La Fortaleza
P.O. Box 9020082
San Juan, PR 00902-0082
Phone: 787/721-7000
Fax: 787/721-5072
http://www.fortaleza.pr.gov

Rhode Island
Office of Governor Gina Raimondo
State House
Providence, RI 02903
Phone: 401/222-2080
Fax: 401/222-8096
http://www.governor.state.ri.us

South Carolina
Office of Governor Henry McMaster
1205 Pendleton Street
Columbia, SC 29201
Phone: 803/734-2100
Fax: 803/734-5167
https://governor.sc.gov/Pages/default.aspx

South Dakota
Office of Governor Dennis Daugaard
500 East Capitol Street
Pierre, SD 57501
Phone: 605/773-3212
Fax: 605/773-4711
http://sd.gov/governor/

Tennessee
Office of Governor Bill Haslam
Tennessee State Capitol
Nashville, TN 37243-0001
Phone: 615/741-2001
Fax: 615/532-9711
https://www.state.tn.us/governor/

Texas
Office of Governor Greg Abbott
P.O. Box 12428
Austin, TX 78711
Phone: 512/463-2000
Fax: 512/463-5571
https://gov.texas.gov

Utah
Office of Governor Gary R. Herbert
Utah State Capitol
Suite 200
Salt Lake City, UT 84114
Phone: 801/538-1000
Fax: 801/538-1557
https://www.utah.gov/governor/

Vermont
Office of Governor Phil Scott
109 State Street
Pavilion Office Building
Montpelier, VT 05609
Phone: 802/828-3333
Fax: 802/828-3339
http://governor.vermont.gov

Virgin Islands
Office of Governor Kenneth Mapp
Government House, 21-22 Kongens Gade
Charlotte Amalie
St. Thomas, VI 00802
Phone: 340/774-0001
Fax: 340/693-4374
https://www.vi.gov/governor.html

Virginia
Office of Governor Terry McAuliffe
State Capitol
Third Floor
Richmond, VA 23219
Phone: 804/786-2211
Fax: 804/371-6351
https://www.governor.virginia.gov

Washington
Office of Governor Jay Inslee
Office of the Governor
P.O. Box 40002
Olympia, WA 98504-0002
Phone: 360/902-4111
Fax: 360/753-4110
https://www.governor.wa.gov

West Virginia
Office of Governor Jim Justice
1900 Kanawha Street
Charleston, WV 25305
Phone: 304/558-2000
https://governor.wv.gov/Pages/default.aspx

Wisconsin
Office of Governor Scott Walker
115 East State Capitol
Madison, WI 53707
Phone: 608/266-1212
Fax: 608/267-8983
https://walker.wi.gov

Wyoming
Office of Governor Matthew Mead
State Capitol Building
Room 124
Cheyenne, WY 82002
Phone: 307/777-7434
Fax: 307/632-3909
http://governor.wyo.gov

National Governors Association
© copyright 2015.
All Right Reserved.
Phone: (202) 624-5300
Fax: (202) 624-5313

HOW TO CONTACT YOUR STATE REPRESENTATIVES

A GUIDE TO CONTACTING YOUR REPRESENTATIVE IS AVAILABLE AT:
https://bebusinessed.com/congress-fax-numbers/h

This guide, posted on the BEBUSINESSED website, includes an interactive map, which allows you to click on your state or type in your postal code abbreviation in an alphabetical list. You'll then see the names, pictures, fax numbers, phone numbers and e-mail addresses for all of the members of the U.S. Congress in your state.

CHAIN DRUG STORE CONTACT INFORMATION

CVS HEALTH CAREMARK

Customer Support Center
One CVS Drive
Woonsocket, RI 02895
http://cvshealth.com

Main: (401) 765-1500
Toll Free: (800) 746-7287

E mail: customercare@cvs.com

EXECUTIVE CONTACTS:

Kevin Hourican
Executive Vice President, CVS Health and President CVS Pharmacy
Customer Support Center
One CVS Drive
Woonsocket, RI 02895
Kevin.Hourican@cvshealth.com

Prem Shah, Pharm D
Executive Vice President Specialty Pharmacy
CVS Health
PremShah@cvshealth.com

Papatya Tankut, Rph
Vice President Pharmacy Affairs, CVS Health
Papatya.Tankut@cvshealth.com

WALGREENS

Main office
Walgreens Boots Alliance, Inc.
108 Wilmot Road
Deerfield, IL 60015

For general inquiries, please contact:
USA, +1 (847) 315-3700
International, +44 (0) 1932 870 550
-Walgreens.com Inquiries: 1-877-250-5823;
-Store Inquiries:1-800-WALGREENS or 1-800-925-4733;
-Corporate Inquiries: 1-847-914-2500;
-Customer Relations: 1-800-925-4733, option 4.

EXECUTIVE CONTACTS:

Richard Ashworth
President, Pharmacy and Retail Operations
richard.ashworth@walgreens.com

Alex Gourlay
Co-chief operating officer for Walgreens Boots Alliance
alex.gourlay@walgreens.com

David Barber
Marketing Divisional Vice President
david.barber@walgreens.com

Michael Darer
VP of Customer and Commercial Insights
michael.darer@walgreens.com

WALMART

702 SW 8th St
Bentonville, AR 72716
www.walmart.com

Main: (479) 273-4000
Toll Free: (800) 925-6278

EXECUTIVE CONTACTS:

Additional contact info for Walmart Executive Office: executive.communications@wal-mart.com

Walmart Executive Escalations:CACSSEE@wal-mart.com

Judith McKenna
Executive Vice President and Chief Operating Officer, Walmart U.S
702 SW 8th St
Bentonville, AR 72716
Judith.McKenna@wal-mart.com

Greg Foran
President and Chief Executive Officer of Walmart U.S.
702 SW 8th St
Bentonville, AR 72716
Greg.Foran@wal-mart.com

Doug McMillon
President and CEO, Wal-Mart Stores, Inc.
702 SW 8th St
Bentonville, AR 72716
Doug.McMillon@wal-mart.com

RITE AID

30 Hunter Lane
Camp Hill, PA 17011

Phone:
1-800-748-3243
(717)761-2633

Web
www.riteaid.com

All customer support contacts are listed on their website. Customer
must fill out an online contact form to be directed to the proper department.

EXECUTIVE CONTACTS:

John T. Standley Chairman and Chief Executive Officer

Kermit Crawford President and Chief Operating Officer

Darren Karst Senior Executive Vice President, Chief Financial Officer, and Chief Administrative Officer

Bryan Everett Chief Operating Officer of Rite Aid Stores

Jocelyn Konrad Executive Vice President, Pharmacy

BIBLIOGRAPHY

Alter, Adam. 2017. *Irresistible: the Rise of Addictive Technology and the Business of Keeping Us Hooked.* New York, NY: Penguin Press.

American Journal of Pharmaceutical Education. 2007. "ncbi.nim.nih.gov." *PMC US National Library of Medicine, National Institutes of Health.* PMCID: PMC1959208. August 15. Accessed July 27, 2017. https://www.ncbi.nlm.nih.gov/pmc/articles/PMC1959208/.

American Pharmacists Association. 2017. *Pharmacy Based Immunization Delivery 14th Edition.* Edited by Sue M. Weedon. Vers. 14. American Pharmacists Association. July 15. Accessed July 10, 2017. www.pharmacist.com/pharmacy-based-immunization-delivery.

Andrews, Michelle. 2017. "NPR." *Shots: Health News from NPR.* April 12. Accessed July 18, 2017. http://www.npr.org/sections/health-shots/2017/04/12/523335954/what-happens-to-a-congressmans-health-insurance-if-obamacare-goes-down.

Boston Globe. 2016. "the Boston Globe." June 30. Accessed August 17, 2017. https://www.bostonglobe.com/metro/2016/06/30/cvs-pays-million-settle-federal-probe-that-found-pharmacists-filled-forged-prescriptions/btKqNm4tYmglO3s8qm8V3I/story.html.

Chicago Tribune. 2017. "Chicago Tribune." January 20. Accessed August 17, 2017.

http://www.chicagotribune.com/business/ct-walgreens-discount-settlement-0121-biz-20170120-story.html.

—. 2017. "Chicago Tribune." January 24. Accessed August 23, 2017. http://www.chicagotribune.com/news/watchdog/druginteractions/ct-drug-interactions-illinois-pharmacies-rauner-met-20170124-story.html.

—. 2017. "ChicagoTribune." *chicagotribune.com.* February 7. Accessed July 26, 2017. http://www.chicagotribune.com/news/watchdog/druginteractions/ct-drug-interactions-flowers-pharmacy-20170207-story.html.

CNN. 2012. "CNN." *cnn.com.* April 20. Accessed August 17, 2017. http://www.cnn.com/2012/04/20/health/walgreens-prescription-settlement/index.html?hpt=hp_bn12.

Crain's. 2014. "Crain's Chicago Business." August 19. Accessed August 17, 2017. http://www.chicagobusiness.com/article/20140819/NEWS07/140819837/golden-exits-big-payday-for-departing-walgreen-execs.

CVS. 2010. "CVS Pharmacy Business Metrics." July. Accessed July 10, 2017. https://www.google.com/url?sa=t&rct=j&q=&esrc=s&source=web&cd=4&ved=0ahUKEwi-gPepx4HVAhWrzIMKHcHeDWQQFgg8MAM&url=http%3A%2F%2Fwww.documentcloud.org%2Fdocuments%2F472510-250510-rx-tg.html&usg=AFQjCNFh24F6GppuHG9toi41FOcRo_lU6g.

CVS, Delores V. Wigger v., and 2:15-CV-01122-DCN-MGB. 2014. "pharmacist steve.com." Accessed August 23, 2017. http://www.pharmaciststeve.com/wp-content/uploads/2015/10/cvslawsuit10212015.pdf.

Dollarhide, Adrian W., Thomas Rutledge, Matthew B. Weinger, Erin Stucky Fisher, Sonia Jain, Tanya Wolfson, and Timothy R. Dresselhaus. 2013. "Journal for Healthcare Quality." *Research Gate.* Edited by Dr. P.H. Maulik Joshi. Wolters Kluwer. March 29. Accessed July 6, 2017. https://www.researchgate.net/profile/Thomas_Rutledge/publication/236102371_A_Real-Time_Assessment_of_Factors_Influencing_Medication_Events/links/55229feb0cf2f9c130531ecd.pdf.

Dowell D, Haegerich TM, Chou R. 2016. "CDC." *cdc.gov.* March 18. Accessed August 19, 2017. https://www.cdc.gov/mmwr/volumes/65/rr/rr6501e1.htm#B1_down.

Drug Policy Alliance. 2017. "Drug Policy." *Drug Policy.org.* Accessed August 25, 2017. http://www.drugpolicy.org/facts/new-solutions-drug-policy/brief-history-drug-war-0.

Drug Topics. 2015. November 4. Accessed August 10, 2017. http://drugtopics.modernmedicine.com/drug-topics/news/pharmacy-staffing-levels-can-threaten-patient-lives?utm_source=TrendMD&utm_medium=cpc&utm_campaign=Drug_Topics_TrendMD_0.

—. 2014. "drug topics." *drug topics modern medicine.com.* Edited by Editor by Mark Lowery. June 12. Accessed August 17, 2017. http://drugtopics.modernmedicine.com/drugtopics/content/tags/jeremy-hoven/court-upholds-walgreens-firing-pharmacist-using-handgun.

—. 2015. "Drug Topics." *modern medicine.* Edited by Julianne Stein. Advanstar. July 22. Accessed August 10, 2017. http://drugtopics.modernmedicine.com/drug-topics/news/who-blame-pharmacy-mistakes.

—. 2016. "Drug Topics." October 10. Accessed August 10, 2017. http://drugtopics.modernmedicine.com/drug-topics/news/keys-minimizing-prescription-drug-errors.

—. 2015. "Drug Topics DT Blog." Edited by Julianne Stein. Modern Medicine. August 26. Accessed August 10, 2017. http://drugtopics.modernmedicine.com/drug-topics/news/pharmacists-write-part-2-why-mistakes-happen?page=0,1.

—. 2011. "Drug Topics Magazine." *Drug Topics at Modern Medicine.com.* Edited by Julianne Stein. Advanstar Publications. May 10. Accessed July 29, 2017. http://drugtopics.modernmedicine.com/drug-topics/content/dear-drugmonkey.

—. 2016. "Drug Topics Modern Medicine." *drugtopics.modernmedicine.com.* Edited by Mark Lowery. Advanstar Publications. January 29. Accessed August 3, 2017. http://drugtopics.modernmedicine.com/drug-topics/news/walmart-ordered-pay-pharmacist-31-million-wrongful-termination?page=0,1.

—. 2015. "Drug Topics Voice of the Pharmacist." *Modern Medicine.* Modern Medicine Advanstar. February 27. Accessed August 3, 2017. http://drugtopics.modernmedicine.com/drugtopics/news/second-ala-pharmacist-wins-age-discrimination-lawsuit-against-cvs?page=full.

—. 2015. "Drug Topics Voices." *Drug Topics Modern Medicine.* November 10. Accessed July 20, 2017. http://drugtopics.modernmedicine.com/drug-topics/news/drug-topics-voices-11-10-2015?utm_source=TrendMD&utm_medium=cpc&utm_campaign=Drug_Topics_TrendMD_0.

Drug Topics- Voice of the Pharmacist. 2017. "Drug Topics." *modernmedicine.com.* Edited by Julianne Stein. Accessed August 23, 2017. http://drugtopics.modernmedicine.com/.

Drug Topics, Dennis Miller Rph. 2016. "Drug Topics." Edited by Julianne Stein. February 2016. Accessed August 10, 2017. http://drugtopics.modernmedicine.com/drug-topics/news/pharmacists-and-cognitive-dissonance.

Drug Topics, The Cynical Pharmacist. 2015. "Drug Topics, Modern Medicine." Advanstar Publications. September 2. Accessed August 8, 2017. http://drugtopics.modernmedicine.com/drug-topics/news/close-pharmacy?page=full&utm_source=TrendMD&utm_medium=cpc&utm_campaign=Drug_Topics_TrendMD_0.

Drugwatch. 2016. "drugwatch.com." Accessed August 22, 2017. https://www.drugwatch.com/manufacturer/#about-big-pharma.

Federal Election Commission. 2017. "Reports Image Index for Committee ID C00160770." *FEC Website.* Accessed July 27, 2017. http://docquery.fec.gov/cgi-bin/fecimg/?C00160770.

Forbes. 2014. November 26. Accessed August 10, 2017. https://www.forbes.com/sites/nickmorrison/2014/11/26/the-myth-of-multitasking-and-what-it-means-for-learning/.

—. 2013. "Forbes.com." Contributor Bruce Jepsen. February 8. Accessed August 8, 2017. https://www.forbes.com/sites/brucejapsen/2013/02/08/how-flu-shots-became-big-sales-booster-for-walgreen-cvs/#5641869271ce.

Fortune. 2015. "Fortune.com." August 6. Accessed August 17, 2017. http://fortune.com/2015/08/06/highest-ceo-worker-pay-ratio/.

Frank, Jeffrey. 2017. "The New Yorker." *Daily Comment.* January 17. Accessed July 18, 2017. http://www.newyorker.com/news/daily-comment/on-health-care-well-have-what-congress-is-having.

Glassdoor. 2011. "Glass Door." *CVS Health Overworked and Understaffed.* February 7. Accessed August 17, 2017. https://www.glassdoor.com/Reviews/Employee-Review-CVS-Health-RVW802425.htm.

Good Jobs First. 2017. "Good Jobs First." *Violations Tracker.* Accessed August 17, 2017. http://violationtracker.goodjobsfirst.org/parent/.

Good Morning America. 2011. "sommerspc.com." *Sommers Schwartz Law Offices.* Sommers Schwartz Law Offices. September 12. Accessed August 12, 2017. https://www.sommerspc.com/videos/abc-good-morning-america-jeremy-hoven-wrongful-termination/.

Hannah Family, in the second year of her PhD studies at the University's Department of Pharmacy & Pharmacology, will be working in a research team led by Dr Jane Sutton and supported by Professor Marjorie Weiss. 2012. "Bath ac UK." *University of Bath.* February 2012. Accessed July 6, 2017. http://www.bath.ac.uk/news/2012/02/27/pharmacists-workload/.

Harper's. 2016. "Legalize It All How to win the war on drugs." *Harpers Magazine.* April. Accessed August 25, 2017. https://harpers.org/archive/2016/04/legalize-it-all/.

HHS. 2015. "Dept of Health and Human Services Public Access." March 1. Accessed August 10, 2017. https://www.ncbi.nlm.nih.gov/pmc/articles/PMC3805762/ .

—. 2013. "Health and Human Services Public Access." April 12. Accessed August 10, 2017. https://www.ncbi.nlm.nih.gov/pmc/articles/PMC3624990/ .

HHS Public Access. 2010. February 11. Accessed August 10, 2017. https://www.ncbi.nlm.nih.gov/pmc/articles/PMC3052977/ .

HHS.gov. 2009. 16 January. Accessed 17 August, 2017. https://www.hhs.gov/hipaa/for-professionals/compliance-enforcement/examples/CVS/index.html.

Hussar, Daniel. 2014. *The Pharmacist Activist.* April. Accessed July 10, 2017. http:\\thepharmacistactivist.com.

Indeed.com. 2015. February 9. Accessed August 15, 2017. https://www.indeed.com/cmp/Walmart/reviews?fcountry=ALL&fjobtitle=Pharmacy+Manager&ftopic=jobsecadv.

n.d. "Indiana General Assembly Archive." *in.gov.*

Indiana General Assembly. 2012. "Indiana General Assembly Archives." *in.gov.* March 9. Accessed July 29, 2017. http://www.in.gov/apps/lsa/session/billwatch/billinfo?year=2012&request=getBill&docno=407#latest_info.

Info Wars. 2012. "Info Wars." *infowars.com.* September 24. Accessed July 26, 2017. https://www.infowars.com/pharmacies-profit-from-dangerous-flu-shot-disrupt-medical-records/.

Institute for Safe Medication Practices (ISMP). 2012. "ISMP Newsletter." *A Non Profit Organization Educating the Healthcare Community About Safe Medication Practices.* September 6. Accessed July 7, 2017. http://www.ismp.org/Newsletters/acutecare/showarticle.aspx?id=30.

Jim Plagakis. 2011. "ehealthforum.com." *E Health Forum.* July 11. Accessed August 3, 2017. http://ehealthforum.com/blogs/jpgakis/let-s-support-kelly-hoots-in-the-cvs-drama-b19250.html.

Joe and Teresa Graedon, People's Pharmacy. n.d. *SunSentinel.* http:.

John Russel, Reporter. 2014. "INDYSTAR part of the USA Today Network." March 30. Accessed July 10, 2017. http://www.indystar.com/story/news/politics/2014/03/30/pharmacy-boards-actions-raise-questions-ethics-patient-privacy-safety/7088079/.

Johnson, Parris and. n.d. "slideshare." *slideshare.net*. https://www.slideshare.net/rfvasquezr/the-history-of-pain-medicine.

Kristy Malacos, MS, CPhT. 2016. "Pharmacy Times." June 16. Accessed July 10, 2017. http://www.pharmacytimes.com/publications/issue/2016/june2016/pharmacy-technician-regulation.

LaMendola, Bob. 1998. October 25. Accessed July 6, 2017. articles.sun-sentinel.com.

Linkedin. 2017. "Linked In." August 15. Accessed August 15, 2017. https://www.linkedin.com/in/christopher-hall-41b96129.

Los Angeles Times. 2000. "articles at La times." Los Angeles Times. February 2000. Accessed August 10, 2017. http://articles.latimes.com/2000/feb/27/news/mn-3125.

Mass.gov Health and Human Services Department. 2017. Accessed August 10, 2017. http://www.mass.gov/eohhs/gov/departments/dph/programs/hcq/dhpl/pharmacy/medication-error-prev/med-error-study/results/.

Members Present: Kim Caldwell (TX), chair, Joseph Adams (LA), Vernon H. Benjamin (IA), Amy Buesing (NM), James T. DeVita (MA), Randall Knutsen (CO), Paul Limberis (CO), et al. n.d. "Report of the Task Force on Continuous Quality Improvement, Peer Review, and Inspecting for Patient Safety." https://nabp.pharmacy/wp-content/uploads/2016/07/07-08TF-CQI.pdf.

Members Present: Task Force on Workload Systems John D. Taylor, Chair (FL), SuAnn M. Bond (WA), Jr. (TX) Fred S. Brinkley, Executive Committee Liaison, (OH) Bonnie

Wallner (DE). Others Present: Jerry Moore, NABP Executive Director Carmen A. Catizone, and NABP Staff. Introduction: Janice Teplitz. 1995. "National Association of Boards of Pharmacy." *NABP* . Edited by NATIONAL ASSOCIATION OF BOARDS OF PHARMACY • (P) 847/391-4406 • (F) 847/391-4502 • www.nabp.net. September. Accessed July 6, 2017. https://nabp.pharmacy/wp-content/uploads/2016/07/TF-Workload-Systems_AM92_1996.pdf.

Mirriam Webster Dictionary. 2017. "Mirriam Webster Online." Accessed July 28, 2017. https://www.merriam-webster.com/dictionary/prostitute.

NABP. 2001. "1996 Report of the Task Force on Workload Systems." *1996 Report of the Task Force on Workload Systems.* February 1. Accessed July 6, 2017. https://nabp.pharmacy/1996-report-of-the-task-force-on-workload-systems/.

—. 2001. "1998 Task Force on Workload Systems February 1, 2001 ." February 1. Accessed July 6, 2017. https://nabp.pharmacy/1998-task-force-on-workload-systems/.

—. 2017. "NATIONAL ASSOCIATION OF BOARDS OF PHARMACY." *NABP.* Edited by IL 60056 Mailing Address: NABP 1600 Feehanville Dr Mount Prospect. Accessed August 4, 2017. https://nabp.pharmacy/boards-of-pharmacy/.

NIH. 2012. "PubMed.gov." February 24. Accessed August 10, 2017. https://www.ncbi.nlm.nih.gov/pubmed/22775522.

PAC, FEC/CVS CAREMARK. 2017. Accessed July 27, 2017. https://www.fec.gov/data/committee/C00327916/.

Pardo, B. 2017. "Addiction, doi 10.1111/add.13741." Vers. doi:10.1111. John Wiley & Sons, Ltd. February 8. Accessed August 19, 2017. http://onlinelibrary.wiley.com/doi/10.1111/add.13741/abstract.

Penn Live.com. 2013. "Penn Live." *Penn Live.com.* July 22. Accessed July 29, 2017. http://www.pennlive.com/midstate/index.ssf/2013/07/ex-cvs_pharmacist_claims_he_wa.html.

Pharmacist workload and pharmacy characteristics associated with the dispensing of potentially clinically important drug-drug interactions Daniel C. Malone, Jacob Abarca, Grant H. Skrepnek, John E. Murphy, Edward P. Armstrong, Amy J. Grizzle, Rick A. Rehfeld, Raymond L. Woosley. 2007. "Th University of Arizona." *Arizona Commerce Authority Board of Regents, Arizona's Public Universities.* May. https://arizona.pure.elsevier.com/en/publications/pharmacist-workload-and-pharmacy-characteristics-associated-with-.

Pharmacy Times. 2017. April 21. Accessed August 10, 2017. http://www.pharmacytimes.com/news/recent-pharmacy-robbery-statistics.

—. 2016. "Pharmacy Times ." *Pharmacy TImes.* June 2016. Accessed July 29, 2017. http://www.pharmacytimes.com/publications/issue/2016/june2016/pharmacy-technician-regulation.

—. 2017. "Pharmacy Times ." *Pharmacy Times Online.* January 9. Accessed August 3, 2017. http://www.pharmacytimes.com/association-news/daniel-a-hussar-named-2017-remington-honor-medal-recipient-highest-honor-in-pharmacy.

Phd, Adam J Fein. 2008. "Drug Channels." *Expert insights on Pharmaceutical Economics and the Drug Distribution System.* Edited by Adam J Fein. February 13. Accessed July 7, 2017. http://www.drugchannels.net/2008/02/dark-side-of-pharmacy-efficiency.html.

Phd, Daniel Hussar. 2008. "The Pharmacist Activist." *The Pharmacist Activist Newsletter.* Edited by Philadelphia College of Pharmacy Daniel Hussar Phd. February . Accessed July 7, 2017. http://www.pharmacistactivist.com/2008/pdfs/February_2008.pdf.

Plagakis, Jim. 2012. "E Health Forum." *ehealthforum.com/blogs.* June 8. Accessed August 1, 2017. http://ehealthforum.com/blogs/jpgakis/a-female-wag-pharmacist-and-wag-shareholder-lets-loose-b29477.html.

PRESS, JOHN HENDREN | ASSOCIATED. 2000. "Los Angeles Times." *LA Times Web Page.* Februarty 27. Accessed July 6, 2017. http://articles.latimes.com/2000/feb/27/news/mn-3125.

Publication, The Pharmaceutical Journal/A Royal Pharmaceutical Society. 2009. Jun 12. Accessed July 6, 2017. http://www.pharmaceutical-journal.com/news-and-analysis/news/errors-are-just-one-aspect-of-the-workload-problem/10966945.article.

PubMed. 2011. "PubMed.gov." *ncbi nim nih . gov.* Jul:29(3):33,36-9 Bull Anesth Hist. 2011. July 29. Accessed August 25, 2017. https://www.ncbi.nlm.nih.gov/pubmed/22849210.

Rat-King, Katharina Fritsch:. 1993. "Dia Art program/exhibitions." *Dia Art* . April 15. Accessed August 23, 2017. https://www.diaart.org/program/exhibitions-projects/katharina-fritsch-rat-king-exhibition.

Reddit. 2014. "reddit.com." Accessed August 24, 2017. https://www.reddit.com/r/pharmacy/comments/1vnjbg/pharmacist_kill_themselves_more_than_any_other/.

Reporters, Ray Long and Sam Roe-Contact. 2017. "Chicago Tribund." *Chicago Tribune.* Edited by Publisher and Editor in Cheif R Bruce Dold. IL 60611 312 222-3232 Chicago Tribune 435 N. Michigan Ave. Chicago. February 7. Accessed July 6, 2017. whttp://www.chicagotribune.com/news/watchdog/druginteractions/ct-drug-interactions-flowers-pharmacy-20170207-story.html.

Robert Mabee, Rph, JD, MBA. n.d. *Drug Topics* .

Rosenfeld, Jonathan. 2015. "Rosenfeld Injury Lawyers." *Personal Injury News and Developments.* June 1. Accessed July 6, 2017. https://www.rosenfeldinjurylawyers.com/news/a-proactive-approach-to-reducing-pharmacy-errors/.

Rph, Dennis Miller. 2015. "Drug Topics." Edited by Julianne Stein. August 5. Accessed August 10, 2017. http://drugtopics.modernmedicine.com/drug-topics/news/pharmacy-mistakes-part-3-state-bops-and-public-safety.

Steve Ariens, pharmaciststeve.com. n.d. "Pharmacist Steve." *pharmacist steve.com.*

Systems, Nabp Task Force on Workload. 1998. Jan 23 24. Accessed July 6, 2017. https://nabp.pharmacy/wp-content/uploads/2016/07/TFWorkloadSystems_AM94_Jan 1998.pdf.

The Chicago Tribune. 2016. "The Chicago Tribune." *chicagotribune.com.* December 15. Accessed July 27, 2017. http://www.chicagotribune.com/news/watchdog/druginteractions/ct-drug-interactions-pharmacy-met-20161214-story.html.

The New Yorker. 2014. May 7. Accessed August 10, 2017. http://www.newyorker.com/science/maria-konnikova/multitask-masters.

The Purdue Pharmacist . 2012. "The Purdue Pharmacist ." Spring Summer. Accessed August 12, 2017.

TODAY, KEVIN MCCOY and USA. 2008. "ABC NEWS.COM." December 30. Accessed July 10, 2017. http://abcnews.go.com/Business/story?id=6552337&page=1.

Topics, Drug. 2015. September 11. Accessed August 10, 2017. http://drugtopics.modernmedicine.com/drug-topics/news/pharmacist-error-rate-rises-workload-climbs?page=full.

Tribune, Chicago. 2016. "The Chicago Tribune." *chicagotribune.com.* May 11. Accessed August 17, 2017. http://www.chicagotribune.com/business/ct-cvs-pharmacists-contract-0511-biz-20160510-story.html.

U.S. News Online. 1996. "Health News Review.org." *U.S. News Online 08/26/96.* August 26. Accessed July 26, 2017. https://www.healthnewsreview.org/wp-content/uploads/2017/01/DangerattheDrugstore10.doc.pdf.

University of Arizona. 25. University of Arizona Health Sciences Center. April 2007. Accessed August 10, 2017. https://www.sciencedaily.com/releases/2007/04/070424130317.htm.

University of Cincinnati. 2001. Accessed August 10, 2017. http://www.angelo.edu/faculty/kschell/downloads/Grasha_Schell2001.pdf.

USA Today. 2013. "usa today." *usa today.com.* June 11. Accessed August 17, 2017. https://www.usatoday.com/story/news/nation/2013/06/11/walgreens-drug-oxycodone-license-80-million/2412451/.

V.M. Lea, S.A. Corlett, R.M. Rodgers. n.d. "Research In Social and Administrative Pharmacy." *Medway School of Pharmacy Universities of Kent and Greenwich , Chatham, Kent, United Kingdo.* http://www.rsap.org/article/S1551-7411(14)00144-2/fulltext.

Washington State Quality Assurance Commission. 2015. "Washington State Government Website." *Department of Health Wa.gov.* March 9. Accessed July 29, 2017. http://www.doh.wa.gov/Portals/1/Documents/2300/2015/RulesOtherStates.pdf.

Wikipedia. 2017. "wikipedia." *Wilipedia.* August 16. Accessed August 19, 2017. https://en.wikipedia.org/wiki/Prescription_monitoring_program.

—. 2017. "wikipedia." Accessed August 22, 2017. https://en.wikipedia.org/wiki/Rat_king.

APPENDIX

PHARMACY BLOGS, WEBSITES, AND FACEBOOK PAGES

And You Wonder Why Your Pharmacist Never Smiles
http://stupidthingsnpeople.blogspot.com/

The Angry Pharmacist
https://www.theangrypharmacist.com/

The Blonde Pharmacist
http://www.theblondepharmacist.com/blog

Bulldog Pharmacist http://bulldogpharmacist.blogspot.com

Crazy Rx Man http://crazyrxman.blogspot.com/

CVS-Profit$ Over Patients$ http://cvs-greed.blogspot.com/

DEA Chronicles http://deachronicles.quarles.com/h

DEA Sucks http://www.deasucks.com/index.htmh

Do Not Dispense https://donotdispense.wordpress.com/h

Drug Monkey http://drugmonkey.blogspot.com/

Drug Topics http://drugtopics.modernmedicine.com/drug-topics/category/drug-topics/blog

Drugs R Phun http://mandyiscool.blogspot.com/

The Digital Apothecaryhttp://www.thedigitalapothecary.com/

Fast Food Pharmacyhttp://fastfoodpharmacy.blogspot.com/

The Frantic Pharmacist http://franticpharmacist.blogspot.com/

Guerrilla Pharmacist https://www.facebook.com/theguerrillapharmacist/

Jim Plagakis https://jimplagakis.com/h

Pandemic of Denial http://pandemicofdenial.com

Painpedia http://pain.wikidot.com/h

Painkiller Law Blog http://www.painkillerlaw.com/painkiller-law-blog/

Pharmacy Roulette https://www.facebook.com/PharmacyRouletteYouBetYourLife

Pill Pusher Chronicles http://pillpusher.blogspot.com/h

Pharmacist Activist http://www.pharmacistactivist.com/

Pharmacy Chick http://pharmacychick.com/

Pharmacy Slave http://pharmacyslave.blogspot.com/

Pharmacist Jamie http://pharmacistjamie.com/

Pharmacist Steve http://pharmaciststeve.com

Pharmacy Mike http://pharmacymike.blogspot.com/

Pharmacy God http://pharmacygod.blogspot.com/

Pharm Barbie http://pharmbarbie.blogspot.com/

Pharmdblogger http://pharmdblog.blogspot.com/

The Phrustrated Pharmacist http://tphrph.blogspot.com/h

Pissed Pharmacist http://pissedpharmacist.blogspot.com/

Slaves for Walgreens
http://slavesforwalgreens.blogspot.com/

Some Pharmacy Guy
http://somepharmacyguy.blogspot.com/

Soul Sucking Pharmacy
http://soulsuckingpharmacy.blogspot.com/

The Cynical Pharmacist
http://thecynicalpharmacist.blogspot.com/h

The Honest Apothecary
http://www.thehonestapothecary.com/

The Law of Compounding
www.lawofcompoundingmedications.com

The Ole' Apothecary
https://theoleapothecary.wordpress.com/

The Redheaded Pharmacist
www.theredheadedpharmacist.com/

ARTICLES ABOUT PHARMACIST WORKLOAD

"Overwork Threatens Druggists Accuracy (Los Angeles Times 2000)

"Pharmacists write in, Part 2: Why mistakes happen" (Drug Topics 2015)

"Who is to Blame for Pharmacy Mistakes (Drug Topics 2015)

"Pharmacy Mistakes, Part 3: State BOP's and public safety" (Drug Topics 2015)

"Pharmacists and Cognitive Dissonance" (Drug Topics 2016)

"Keys to Minimizing Prescription Drug Errors" (Drug Topics 2016)

"Pharmacy Staffing levels Can Threaten Patient Lives" (Drug Topics 2015)

"Pharmacist Error Rate Rises as Workload Climbs" (Topics 2015, Drug Topics 2015)

Pharmacists Workload Contributes to Errors" (University of Arizona 25)

Medication Error Study, Mass.gov Health and Human Services (Mass.gov Health and Human Services Department 2017)

"Community Pharmacists' Subjective Workload and Perceived Task Performance: a Human Factors Approach" (HHS 2013)

"The Association of Subjective Workload Dimensions on Quality of Care and Pharmacist Quality of Work Life" (HHS 2015)

"The Myth of Multitasking and What it Means for Learning" (Forbes 2014)

"Multitask Masters" (The New Yorker 2014)

"Psychosocial Factors, Workload, and Human Error in a Simulated Pharmacy Dispensing Task" (University of Cincinnati 2001)

"Workload and its impact on community pharmacists' job satisfaction and stress: a review of the literature" (NIH 2012)

www.ingramcontent.com/pod-product-compliance
Lightning Source LLC
Chambersburg PA
CBHW071634220526
45469CB00002B/616